HOSPITALITY AND HUMANIZATION AT HOSPITALS

How to make your hospital more human and looks like a hotel!

Adalto Felix de Godoi

DEDICATION

To my wife Daniele, and my daughters Anna Luiza and Gabriela. They make my life full of happiness and rewarding.

To my beloved sisters Neuza Bauries and Nilceia Felix.

To my family, because to belong to a family is still the best part of living in this world.

ACKNOWLEDGMENTS

I would like to say thanks to the hospitals whose images were displayed in this book, my intention was not to advertise their services, but to show how the hospital environment can contribute positively with the patient recovery, with a good administration and people highly interested in changing the world around us – mainly when we more need it. The images materializes the words.

I beg the readers pardon for any mistake or grammar errors committed in this book. As a non-native English speaker, if you find an grammar error it was not intentional.

TABLE OF CONTENTS

INTRODUCTION

A few years ago to talk about some aspects of hospitality, as the introduction of hotel services in hospitals with many doctors and hospital managers was a daunting task, unproductive and sometimes resulted in conflict. There was a lot of resistance to change the hospital environment, to introduce additional services focusing in humanizing the care, as well as the attention directed to the safety and quality of the patient care. Fortunately, today we can find many books written by many authors including doctors, addressing the importance of hospitality, the humanization of hospitals and the positive effects produced by the environment and from the distinguished service. A great and welcome change of mind in the hospital management environment that sees not only the medical treatment as the only path to healing.

Gradually this approach is getting the deserved attention being placed in strategic planning of hospitals that want to differentiate their services, or reposition itself in the health care market. Probably, it will soon become a common practice at most private and public hospitals as happened with hospital certification systems (Accreditation Systems) occurred in recent years in several countries, been considered a differential to many hospitals in several countries which is attracting international patients by the quality and warm attention of their professionals. Being even more auspicious, that mentality also permeates public hospitals with initiatives that require more goodwill and management techniques than necessarily money.

We live in an age where companies from different segments fight fiercely to keep their best and most profitable customers, also to keep their market share obtained often in fierce commercial deals and to grab new customers and new segments already exploited by their competitors. For many, it is often a matter of survival and not just a growth strategy, even in the health care market. In addition, hospitals also need to justify the rising costs of its services to insurers and other clients, and many hospitals does it improving its facilities implementing new services adding value to the service provided.

To remain successful in the market a company must be competitive, constantly innovative and having differentiated products that are attractive to customers, reducing or minimizing the competitors strengths. This is true for almost all market segments, even if it is the health care market, whose satisfaction is derived from the result of a service considered an intangible asset - the health. Like other companies, hospitals in many countries also operate in a competitive environment, where those considered the best hospitals are those which constantly innovate and offer differentiated services that go beyond its core product, which is also a service, the "cure" or the "health".

Until a few years ago, hospitals were known as cold places, avoided when possible, whose image was related more to pain, disease and death than to life. To say to someone that a beloved one was in a hospital was often interpreted as a bad news. In some segments of the society, this same information is now associated with an improvement in the body, an aesthetic plastic surgery or rejuvenating procedure. This new mindset change has occurred after the delivering of the new services in innovative hospitals, which became known as hospitality or hotel services inside hospitals. The successful medical treatment is already considered a commodity, mainly now that a patient can find it anywhere in the world and is the minimum expected from a doctor and a hospital, leading to the question: "what else the hospital can offer to the patient during their treatment?"

Despite the successful models that have emerged in recent years most hospitals has done little to become competitive in the market when the approach is the human part of the medical treatment. Most of them advertise its high-tech equipment and unquestionable protocols, forgetting that a cold ICU (Intensive Care Unit) or the best equipment are not able to replace the warmth of a friendly hug or a family kiss for someone who is dying. Problems of quality, of a poor service and little or no warmth attention provided by the hospital to a considerable number of clients, are leading them to seek treatment in another hospital or abroad. No one cannot ignore that the hospitals clients know what they want and need, and it is not exactly what hospital managers are always interested to offer to their clients.

With the rising costs and demand for healthcare services in recent years, resulted of a greater concern with the people health, the new technologies, the legal matters and the increase of old and new diseases among the population, there is now a portion of customers who require a special attention and are able to pay more to have the best care. Many hospitals seem to face some difficulty in developing a business strategy that addresses this market niche, while others seems to be successful. This differentiation has been perceived as a continuous improvement of care provided to overall clients, adding new services and products to those already offered by the hospital, as hospitality services from the hotel industry, creating an atmosphere that promotes the recovery of the patient with the biggest comfort possible.

This book covers the hospitality management in hospitals and/or healthcare institutions, encouraging them to become competitive against their competitors using successful strategies used in many countries such as the inclusion of luxury and hospitality services. It also covers common problems in the hospital environment as the medical error (malpractice) and failures in the communication and the missing humanization as an indispensable part of the relationship between the hospital and the patient.

Among the objectives of this book it shows the new mentality that permeates hospitals in many countries with hospitality services and new professionals from other industries, which is making the difference, despite certain prejudices and the aversion to innovation in many hospitals. This is complimentary to the medical treatment according with the local laws and regulations, being useful to private, philanthropic, non-governmental and even public hospitals that can benefit from the book's content developing successful strategies with the introduction of hospitality services in their hospitals. Just as occurs in various sectors of the economy adding value to the product or service that the customer buys exceeding its expectations, it can also occur in the health care segment by making a pleasurable experience the treatment and the pursuit of healing in hospitals.

This book also deals with some further issues discussed outside the hospital environment and which deserve the attention of managers and healthcare professionals. It is the care of people of the same sex, errors and malpractices in hospitals, the special needs of different customers, safety and quality of care, among other topics besides presenting the hospitality in hospitals facing the luxury and comfort in some existing cities and countries. What may seem daring today may soon become a routine and a requirement for hospitals wishing to stand out in the market.

Read! If you want to be up to date with what is happening in the world, why many people go to another state or to cross borders to find a better (not always a cheaper) medical treatment abroad and what they find there, and finally some of the best practices we always can learn from. Of course, due to laws and regulations not everything can be applied everywhere, but is a good benchmark to discuss in the next managerial meeting of your hospital. What we cannot forget is that, some facts we use to not consider are nearer than we think... sometimes is the next door. Have a pleasurable reading!

Chapter 1

THE CONCEPT AND DEVELOPMENT OF HOSPITALITY SERVICES AT HOSPITALS

In recent years many books and articles have been written with mentions about the hospitality and a wide range of services and other changes that occurred in the hospital environment around the world, such as beautiful facilities, the sustainability and the concern for patient safety. In many regions these changes focus on the warmth of their social relations with people closer to each other, in others the focus is in the physical structure of the hospital, the design, the protocols and in the quality assurance systems.

In the health care industry the hospitality itself found its own way through differentiated services from the hotel industry improving the wellbeing of patients and visitors during the care, breaking concepts and paradigms by the introduction of products and services previously restricted to hotels, also humanizing the care provided by some health care institutions. The result has turned the hospitality as a synonymous of quality in hospital environments.

The hospitality is as old as the human history as described in numerous books since the prehistoric ages, even in a rudimentary way, to receive, to care and celebrate together are still gregarious characteristics of the human being. The etymology of the words explains the origin of the name hospital. According to BOEGER (2003) the meaning of the Latin word "hóspes" (guest), is the result of the "hospitalis" and "hospitium" words, which in ancient times designated the establishments used to house not only the travelers and pilgrims as well as the disabled and other patients. Usually the same site that hosted travelers, feudal lords, the crusades in the medieval age among others, was also the same place where the wounded and sickness were treated.

The meaning of the word "hospitality" can be found in many dictionaries and comes from the Latin language "hospitalitate" and is defined as "the quality of hospitality, the act of hosting, liberality to guests". Others definitions are "a friendly reception and treatment of guests or strangers", "the disposition of receiving and treating guests and strangers as closers" and other definition from the Latin word "hospitalariu" is "the person which hosts for kindness or charity, friendly person, charitable person". The reader can find other meanings and definitions in many dictionaries with variations in different countries, but with the same basis.

Thus, we can define hospitality as the act of receiving and welcome a visitor, a family member, a friend or a stranger. It means that we give welcome and attention not only to known people regardless of the interests involved. The role of hospitality is crucial, especially in hotels and hospitals due to the ever pressing needs of human beings when they need food, shelter and medical care. The hospitality makes the arrival warmer, rather than simply to meet the needs or desires of a traveler on vacation or a patient in need of hospitalization.

We can find many stories involving the early periods of the human history, covering Biblical times, in the medieval age and mainly with increase of mass travel. There are many biblical references to hospitality in several books, see in the Bible Isaiah 58:7; Joshua 21:13, referencing especially on lodging, Genesis 42:27, 43:21, and many exhortations to the practice of hospitality in the New Testament 1° S. Peter 4:9; Hebrews 13:2; Matthew 25:35,36; 1° Timothy 5:10.

Since the human need for gathering and hunting, eating and feeling heated around fire in caves, as prehistoric drawings shows in the walls, till the most luxurious hotels we have today, at any given time there is record of care and protection among people. In search of food and/or shelter, men traveled migrating or venturing into the unknown and inhospitable regions to better places. Facing dangerous times, the death or greeted by strangers many of them gathered in small villages becoming with time in major cities. With the increase of these migrations and the rising flow of travelers many inns and guesthouses were opened across roads and villages, which allowed to travel more comfortable for individuals, traders and members of the nobility, popularizing the formal and paid hospitality.

The crusades in the medieval age contributed with this scenario due to the need of treatment of the injured in the battles, creating or selecting places and homes designed to treat those in need in the paths or near the sites of their major battles. At that time many diseases and pests have spread easily among people, mainly because of the poor hygiene and inadequate food provision. These sites intended to care and to rehabilitate the sickness and wounded people were the forerunners of our modern hospitals. At that time many residents in the vicinity of the roads and places near the combat field were also obliged by the Crusaders to take care of the sickness, while others did by pity or generosity (Danielou 1966). Over the years there were establishments built specifically for the care of patients as the Hotel of God Hospital in 1772, located in Paris, with 1700 beds which was lately destroyed by a fire.

The hospitality has been currently regarded as something, not always related with medical assistance, which is complimentary to the assistance and adds value to the treatment or cure of a disease in a hospital. The same way the level of hospitality services in the traditional hotel industry is related to the purchasing power of the customer, with option for all budgets even for segments that cannot afford to pay a higher premium, the same is also true in health care where not everyone has access to the best doctors and hospitals, while receiving the treatment they need. In some countries the basics in health care is provided to the people as part of the public service. However, the reality is that the best care, even in those countries with a free healthcare system, will always be provided to those who have access and enough money to pay for it.

This is of great importance in the healthcare system due to the impact the appearance and structure of services provided can have over the patient since his arrival, having the potential to influence positively or negatively the concept of the customer been admitted at the hospital. A greater impact will still be noticed with a warm and helpful welcome and good service, influencing the perception of how fast and effective are the services. When the hospital team does a good job since the patient arrival it facilitates their work with the patient trust in the professionals ability to treat him, reducing the stress not only with the client but also with the family members who accompany him. After all, there is a reason to worry, is the most valuable asset being placed in the hands of these professionals, the patients "life."

Thus, the hospitality is essential within the hospital environment been linked to the process of improvement of the recovery of the patient throughout the time that he is in the hospital. Everyone in the institution will have a decisive role in this process, whether in care as the nursing staff, physiotherapy staff, biomedical professionals and others also providing support to those who directly serve the customer and their families as the administrative and operational departments. Failure at some point of the treatment may lead to a disruption in the excellence of the work done by many other professionals, being unforgivable by the customer and in some circumstances hurting the image of the hospital.

Despite the new concept of care to exist for decades in some hospitals in several countries, it was only in the late eighties that the main exponent of the hospitality inside hospitals, the hotel services, began to receive attention by the media about some hospitals around the world. Some countries like Thailand have been quick to improve the services offered, also creating a structure devoted to the luxury and depersonalization of the hospital, and a complementary structure of care to patients and families before and after the hospitalization comprising hotels, flats, restaurants and including cultural activities. Among the factors that influenced this change, BOEGER cites that:

"A key factor is the patient himself, who began to question and feel the need for the hospital to offer not only the cure or the treatment, as well as safety, comfort and especially their well-being, for your family and visitors." (2003)

GODOI shows other factors than the awareness of customers also was very important to change the customer mindset that enabled the implementation of hospitality and hotels services at hospitals in several countries.

"While some professionals from other fields of knowledge interfere within the process of restructuring the hospital, there are unexpected results especially when questioning obsolete paradigms establishing new truths that become the practice. The hospitality is one of those things when entering the hospital environment with professionals from fields as architecture, tourism, hotel industry, gastronomy among other professions such as designers bringing the similarity between a hospital and a hotel or even with your own home, resulting in one to absorb part of the exclusive services that the other offers. Respecting the appropriate limitations and differences from both places, it is possible to change the cold environment, the smell of hospital and sometimes the sad atmosphere to a new place with natural light, a lively atmosphere, a calm and healthier image, bringing confidence to the patient and his family. The hospital takes on a new profile, that it exists not only to treat patients, but also to produce knowledge, health and quality of life for everyone."(2004)

Due to the awareness of many consumers of health services that the environment can interfere in the healing process, the hospitality has introduced new concepts in hospitals with unthinkable services in the health care industry. Professionals from segments such as hospitality, architecture and gastronomy noticed the structural similarity and the numerous possibilities of adding additional services to medical treatment, resulting in a hospital much more comfortable, functional and above everything more human. Everyone knows how problems with certain members of the staff can interfere in the patient mood, mainly when facing cancer treatment or the risk of death. The hospitality service try to avoid or make the relationship better, helping the patient and his family with everything they need.

BOEGER (2006) defines the hospitality in hospitals as *"[...] all supportive services, which, combined with specific services, provide to the internal and external clients comfort, safety and welfare during the period of hospitalization."* GODOI (2004) does not restrict the benefits of this change only to patients, involving other actors, defining it as *"[...] the introduction of techniques, procedures and hotel services in hospitals with benefits like social, physical, psychological and emotional for patients, families and staff."* The same view is shared by TARABOULSI (2003) which deals with hospitality as a change in the essence of care in hospitals with the introduction of new services and processes in daily treatment, also do not treating the patient as just "another patient".

The hospital-patient relationship has changed significantly in recent years with the continuous improvement of care, greater diagnostic accuracy and reduced time to reach the cure if compared with previous years. These rapid changes occur in other sectors and segments of the economy and could not be different in the health care.

Hospital administrators need to be aware of what happens in the world around them, especially in a segment with a high share of technology and advanced research rapidly reaching the market. Mezomo (1995) makes clear that all these changes, also must reach the hospital environment not only in its physical structure, but mainly on the relationship between the hospital and its patients. He goes further to differentiate human beings from equipments, proposing a steady and growing commitment to the quality aiming failures, errors, infection, and complaints "zero" in the hospitals. After all they are human lives being treated, human lives that need understanding, not just bodies in need of care. Factor of extreme relevance for today's managers is the need to see the patient as a customer whose satisfaction is directly tied to the purchased or recovered product at the hospital, its health and life.

The hospitality introduced a series of new services, not necessarily related to the medical treatment, but with the existing structure and processes within the hospital, changing the mindset of how to treat and to deal with the patient and their families as described below. Several departments were given new assignments or redesigned its flows, while others have been introduced to improve the services available to the customers. These services can fits well in some countries while in others it may seem not necessary, but they are very useful where it was created.

➢ **Reception and Admission:** beyond the maintenance of the patient records, the place is responsible for the patient admission (check-in) and the discharge (check out). Currently, in addition to the pre-admission registration service their job can be done in the patient's room (favoring the mobility) via tablets, laptops or other devices. The multilingual service has become indispensable in top hospitals, as well as all information provided by prospectuses and websites.

➢ **Reservation Department:** the department is normally responsible for scheduling the patient's hospitalization, surgery scheduling, early collection of personal data facilitating the quick admission in the hospital, a previous verification of expenses and special agreements with insurers obtaining prior authorizations. Another activity usually performed is to identify the type of client for distinguished service as a businessman, politicians and personalities.

➢ **Housekeeping:** the department is normally responsible for the hygiene and cleaning of common areas and the inpatient units (rooms), also is responsible for housekeeping, laundry and management of beds in some countries.

➢ **Luggage locker room/department:** it aims to help patients, families or visitants who have baggage and has nowhere to leave, during a visit or either before, during or shortly after discharge from hospital, awaiting for example a flight or a transfer to a hotel.

➢ **Lounge or Waiting room:** shall be large spaces, warm places, very comfortable and if possible illuminated by natural light. The best spaces are in front of plants, flowers or gardens, provided with updated magazines and newspapers, television, etc. with the walls using varied and lively or hot colors, a nice and pleasant music is welcomed. In many hospitals, it's possible to have concerts with violin, piano or other instrument at scheduled times. Usually these concerts are for visitors, caregivers and the public in general, but can also be performed specifically for patients.

➢ **Gift Shop:** very useful for buying last moment gifts or even for a purchase of some personal hygiene objects, underwear forgotten at home or even a souvenir to remember the time in the hospital. They are common in many countries especially in Thailand and in Brazilian hospitals, with some gifts with the hospital logo.

➢ **Bar/Small Kitchen:** exist in many hospitals within rooms/suites or for use of the personnel in the wards. Many top hospitals have a small room inside the suite with microwave and refrigerator making the life easier for caregivers within the apartments. Others hospitals have a Bar for relatives and families celebrate a new baby birth with live transmitting from nursery.

➢ **Flower Shop:** sometimes the visitor have not enough time to buy flowers to bring to the patient, when allowed the entrance of flowers, or left on selected spaces. The flower shop also is useful for visitants, employees and other professionals that want flowers.

➢ **Laundry Service:** some hospitals provide laundry services for patients and caregivers. The service can be offered by the hospital as a business unit within the hospital or in partnership with third parties that may be drawn and delivered at the hospital.

➢ **Restaurant or Bistro:** currently the restaurants of many top hospitals across the world are opened to the outside public that attends even when there is no family in the hospital. With a differentiated menu and high standard service often serve families, physicians and visitors seeking not just a place to dine. Why to go outside and look for a restaurant to have lunch if the hospital can offer it. Many professionals and guests in the hospitals are able to pay more to do not leave the place for a meal.

➢ **Events Department:** the need for constant training and events made many hospitals to build large auditoriums and even convention centers, used for events such as forums, lectures, debates, courses and even conferences. Such spaces does not need to be used only for internal events, been possible to be leased for external events related to the healthcare industry, turning it into a revenue generator for the hospital.

➢ **Gastronomy:** before it was concerned only to provide a food-based diet for patients and in some places for employees. The hospital food use to have a really bad reputation worldwide, despite the importance it has for the patient during his stay. Many hospitals in countries like

Brazil hired chefs from famous restaurants that developed new ways of preparing the hospital food, creating new menus, improving the process and even customizing the patient diet with refined dishes whose taste, appearance and aroma has encouraged patients to eat better. The focus has changed, is taken into account only what the patient cannot eat, instead of the common general prohibition. So, the chef and nutritionists can prepare what the patient like and want to eat having the information only a few hours before the meal been served.

➢ **Suites/Rooms/Apartments:** should have every conceivable comfort including air-conditioning with remote control, mini-bar, flat screen TV, electric beds, and internet access with the possibility of using the personal computer or obtained from the hospital, reclining seats, music, among other benefits as amenities of famous brands in the market. Some hospitals also offer a microwave oven, a bar or eating space and a waiting room in the suites.

➢ **Library:** no matter how unusual it may sound in hospitals, libraries are useful not only to physicians and staff in need of professional books, but also permit the loan of books and periodicals to many patients, family members and caregivers who remain hospitalized for long periods in hospitals. It plays a special role for children spend their time using its time not just watching television.

➤ **Cultural Activities:** presentations of theatre by groups from the hospital or outside groups, visits of clowns (inspired by the Patch Adams movie), individual or group concerts of violin or piano, which has been quite common in hospitals can make the patients and also the staff read more. The presentations can be divided for the children in pediatrics, and to adults in specific places, and even for the staff with an educational thematic or simply focusing on leisure

➤ **Art Gallery:** these are privileged spaces inside hospitals making possible the audience to have contact with the culture (painting, sculptures, etc.) even during the treatment if allowed to the patient leave their suite. Not just the public the relatives and visitors can leave the enclosed space of recovery, the hospital suite, and be in touch with the external environment creating opportunities that go beyond the television and the internet as unique leisure activities, which does little or nothing for the patient to relax.

➤ **Pharmacy or Drugstore:** can exist to facilitating the acquisition of drugs by the patient after the discharge of hospital within the building, serves to support visitors who occasionally also need to purchase medicines and other products.

➤ **Beauty Center:** it is not because someone is under treatment that he or she does not need to look or to feel beautiful. In addition, long hospitalizations require the presence of these professionals to take care of the patient appearance, instead of releasing them to go outside. These services are used in some countries mainly during the stay and before the discharge, not only for patients but also for families, caregivers, visitors and by the staff. Some hospitals prefer to maintain a record of professionals who serves only by appointment.

➤ **Online Visits:** with the mobility problems faced in many cities, travel and inflexible work schedules, it is an essential tool for the patient to receive visits by the internet, and for people who cannot go to the hospital. There are a growing number of hospitals using this tool that will become increasingly useful over time.

➤ **Messaging Service:** when someone cannot visit a person in a hospital or schedule an online visit, the visitor may leave a message, a card or a virtual flower arrangement to the patient. Such services can be provided by the hospital printed or viewed virtually by the patient.

- ➢ **VIP area:** despite the spaces intended for patients and their families, hospitals often receive differentiated persons, as tycoons, famous artists and politicians who need a private space to remain. The *VIP* room allows the patient to not be disturbed unnecessarily, and make possible some services be provided more readily without the public perception. Ideally, have differentiated spaces, tastefully decorated, providing drinks and fruits, computers and other amenities, plus restricted access to ensure the privacy of the person.

- ➢ **Internet Café:** many people in hospitals are away from home and his family, and need to solve administrative problems, send and receive email, print documents, among other needs when they are hospitalized or accompanying someone. Providing a pleasant space for these customer requests prevent troubles to the customers in transit, and becomes a business unit complementing existing services.

- ➢ **Toy Space:** although they are mandatory in public hospitals in some countries like Brazil, they are not always used optimally even in private hospitals. They are essential to reduce the suffering of children whose courage and endurance of pain exceeds that of many adults. Several hospitals that care for disabled children or with cancer have some of the best places, having beside their parent's professionals who accompany them in the brief moments of relief that the games provide.

These new services helped to shape the concept of hospitality in hospitals in several countries of the world, improving the internal environment and diversifying the supply of quality services in these hospitals. Each institution adopts the standard of services that is most appropriate to them, adding some professional or service when they feel it's necessary to humanize the care and also putting these hospitals among the best and most sought when someone needs medical attention and a good hospital. There is no obligation to develop a differentiated service or hiring a new professional, various models established by some hospitals and shown above can be followed with the adequacy of services and expertise of the professionals already in the institution.

To train and to empower employees to carry out new activities will professionalize them by creating new employment opportunities in their future, making them versatile and imbuing in them a sense of gratitude for the company that is investing in their career. If done correctly as a benefit and not as an obligation increasing their duties, the employee usually responds well to the interests of the company. It's not what you ask, it's the way you ask which influences the response of employees. The way some unprepared manager put the need for training to their employees, often makes it seem more a punishment than a professional bonus.

Attention must also be given to the employee uniforms and to the aesthetics, the design and if the clothes fit well are essential for a good presentation with focus on the customer service. There is a clear willingness of many companies to make employees seem really simple staff, while uniforms can be well designed and better represent the role of each professional in the hospital. We all like to be dealing with people well dressed and tidy, and it does not cost much more or are more expensive for the company.

Details such as makeup and hairs are easily noticed in hospitals mainly for women, the employees cannot seem sicker than the customers they help. Some companies can offer a fast course yearly or when possible, or establish partnerships with companies or suppliers of aesthetic beauty products, often at no cost to send a professional and give some useful guidance. This care extends to the men who need care with hair, beards and clothing. Not everybody have the resources or time to pay to such professional services, but when they come to them and teach them to improve appearance, also improve the self-esteem with an obvious positive effects in the professional and personal life of the employee.

Many institutions have created company programs as MBAs aimed at senior management or encouraging the study through short courses. Typically, these investments have been made in higher education and at a technical level, forgetting the need for courses to the operational levels of the company. It is normally the people who have more contact with customers and are the least prepared technically. A cleaning assistant will contact a customer much more than an administrative staff at a managerial level. As discussed in this book, the likelihood of a company loses a customer for a bad service from this professional is higher than the capacity of a senior manager to bring another customer, plus the cost of this new client attraction.

There are a lot of courses on the market that meet all professional needs, and not always to hire consultants to conduct the course in the institution is the best alternative. Partnership with traditional schools allows the employee to suit their schedule with the school, as well as enable the exchange of information and knowledge with other professionals from other institutions, expanding the horizons beyond the doors of the company. Moreover, there is a large amount of distance learning courses that can be made online, depending only to help the employee to overcome difficulty to interact in the virtual environment, or stimulate the managers to see the method with less prejudice and reservations.

The introduction of hospitality services in a hospital or the development of a new mindset through the actions of humanization to the client, meets the need to humanize the care provided by the staff improving too the internal environment and resulting in a modern and efficient structure for everybody. The goal is to make the stay of the patient and his family to be as comfortable and enjoyable as possible, letting the doctor to concern only with the treatment.

Chapter 2

ADMITTANCE, EVALUATION AND PATIENT CARE

Each patient who enters a hospital has different needs and expectations that must be understood individually. The first contact can be tense with a concern about the time that the service will occur, if the professionals who will help are the best professionals, this may even generate some uncertainty and anxiety interfering with the treatment, the medical care and the assistance he or she will receive. Understanding the patient holistically and delivering the adequate care will help him to accept and continue the treatment when leaving the hospital.

So, it is necessary to fully understand more than just the disease that the person has, the staff must understand the feelings of the patient. Many who come are lay people, have cognitive difficulties, face ethnic and cultural barriers, not always adapt easily to the place or fail to establish an effective communication. Moreover, the family or the legal responsible (or the guardian) of the patient must receive due attention and be involved in the treatment as a link between the assistance provided by the hospital and the patient, reducing any barriers that may arise during the treatment of the patient.

As a new situation, it may take some time until the patient and their families to feel familiarized with the facility and structure of the hospital, with the medical terminology and the administrative paperwork necessary to fill. On the other hand, there are patients who seem more comfortable and adapted, but actually know little about the nature of the services later becoming an obstacle to the delivery of care.

To handle all these situations is of great importance that hospitals have mechanisms to ensure that such situations will not go unnoticed. Some institutions, especially those accredited, have a check-list covering the patients' needs and interests of the organization, to see if all procedures and protocols were followed properly. The failure in one may result in the absence of valuable information, or problems may arise later during the care assistance.

A major problem in this world where everyone lives in a hurry and is time-dependent seems to be the little effective communication between people, especially on items that can be left to deal later or there is no urgently need. The feeling that something can be done or told later can have disastrous consequences. When combined with other problems such as the difficulty in understanding, the differences and the many cultural barriers faced within a larger country, the hospital can become an inhospitable environment for patients and health care professionals.

To have an efficient assistance that meets the requirements proposed by the organization or the public authorities the attention is essential in those several stages that begin with the admission of the patient and continue with the transfer to another health service or the safe return to home. It should not end with the discharge of hospital.

Admission and care

When is not a medical emergency, the arrival of the patient may be preceded by a pre-admission form filled by the patient over the internet or from the hospital staff by telephone reducing the waiting time and the tension caused by the fear that something may still not go as planned. In several hospitals around the world the administrative pre-hospitalization process is electronic with the identification of the patient done at the admission and also signing the documents, sometimes already printed in advance. In other hospitals and clinics, an employee call to confirm the admission date, the patient data and contact details sending the forms by email or by mail in advance, so the client can read in advance and bring it signed if desired.

Even with a contact by phone is possible to identify special situations and to check the need to provide a proper service to differentiated patients, like VIP's (Very Important People), dependent of a special accommodation, special people, wheelchair users and older people. Some clerical work can be done in advance as selecting the medical records, results of prior medical evaluation, payments, authorization of procedures can be arranged and communicated to the patient any barriers found. The person can have enough time to solve the problem before arriving at the hospital.

As simple as it sounds, the hospital can become stressful and problematic just when everything should work properly. It is not uncommon during the process of admission emerging new information, new medical fees or additional costs for situations where there is the possibility of non-coverage of a medical procedure from the insurance, and documents to be signed with scary terms. If the check-in at a hotel for leisure or business objective has been minimized to reduce the stress of the guests, the same should occur in hospitals where the "guests" are sick and frail.

Part of this work can be reduced with the availability of so many documents and consent forms as possible on the internet as it occurs in several hospitals across the world even in the United

States, so the patients and their families can read and to question, also reducing printing costs for the hospital.

The technology allows almost all information to be available where the customer is, there is no need to incur in the surprise effect. If the patient has any question or special need, these can be addressed and resolved before the arrival of the patient at the hospital. Mainly because the vast paperwork and documents that need to be signed at a delicate time, when normally the patient and their families are not able to analyze or discuss anything.

Upon arriving to be admitted, the identity is checked, the data updated and verification of information collected prior or by the internet. This reduces the waiting time and intervention by the employee leaving more time to pay attention to other needs of the patient and family. It is interesting to note that in many hospitals the staff are so busy filing reports and with their clerical work that the patient seems to bother them. By reducing the amount of work, is expected to the employees have plenty of time to care for exceptions or for the patients coming from the emergency room.

Some patients have specific needs as a physical, hearing, cognitive or are

8,7% of the U.S. population or more than 24 million of people do not speak English well or have a limited understanding of the language, especially when it comes with the medical terminology.

Source: Joint Commission International

impaired. It should be noticed before, not on the time of arrival. Usually the nursing staff is prepared to deal with these situations. The problem is that not all in the administration teams are, that's why it is important to get this information in advance.

Unfortunately, hospitals seem to give little importance to the training of clerical staff to provide a proper care to patients with special needs, foreign patients or using, for example, sign language. It is critical to have professionals available to handle with these situations and not just to wait a companion of the patient to do this service. There are hospitals that map their employees fluent in foreign and sign languages releasing this information internally for help when there is some need.

With the increasing number of executives and tourists traveling for several reasons and seeking medical treatment in other countries, is increasingly common emergencies occur in major foreign cities worldwide. In addition to communication that needs to be effective and happens in the patient's place in the language or in English/Spanish, considered universal languages, there is the need that all documents be in these languages so the patient can understand what they are signing. The proper assistance should include supplementary information material in different languages and media, such as pictures and letters to attend the hearing impaired and audio to meet the visually impaired. With the technology available today, the hospital can reduce the cost of the material, with storage, recording and printing it to specific situations (on demand) without the generation of additional costs to the institution.

In the hospital daily routine there are critical moments and specific situations in which the employees need training to do a good job. No patient is equal to each other and the attention needs to take it into account, nurses and the administrative staff. Some situations require training to enable frontline staff to treat adequately those customers considered too demanding, high-profile businessmen, public figures and members of the government. There are delicate situations like the death, hospitalization of lonely patients or same-sex couples. In some situations the hospital may have clear protocols and guidelines, and for others what will count is the individual ability of the professional to determine the quality of the care delivered at this critical moment.

Institutionally, the hospital must learn to deal with unusual situations that may occur more frequently in difficult times. Any misplaced comments or improper professional behavior may result in major headaches for the institution. There are situations when the patient designates the partner of the same sex as their legal representative, which is their right in some countries, or when the patient is unconscious, his family refuses to accept the union, and try to restrict its responsibility or the visits of the partner. Are example of situations that the hospital staff will face and have to deal.

In such cases is important to check if there is a legal precedent such as the law allowing or recognizing the stable union of same-sex couples or to adopt children in this kind of relationship. It is up to the hospital managers use common sense if the situation is legal and make the process similar to the others patients not committing the mistake of treating these public differently. With the increasing recognition and respect to the movement so-called Gay, Lesbian, Bisexual and Transgender or otherwise, health care institutions need to adapt and learn to deal with the problems that can occur with the customer service regardless of sexual orientation.

Bad communication is one of the biggest barriers during the interview with the doctors or the hospital staff, the patient and his family may have some difficulty understanding the medical terminology during the process of communication used by the professionals. The forms and documents required to be signed usually have some kind of technical terminology unusual to their daily lives. Although it is easier to ignore or minimize the level of the patient understanding, the hospital managers must notice the importance of to clearly state what some words means and the implications of the signature on each document presented to the patient or his legal representative.

A study conducted by White and Dillow in the United States in 2003 showed that 36% or approximately 87 million American adults have a level of understanding of health terms classified as basic or below basic, and that 88% of adults are not familiar with the most common terms related to health. The cost of problems resulting from this deficiency has been estimated for the U.S. healthcare system as approximately $ 58 billion, and for the economy as a whole the estimate was between $ 106 and $ 236 billion annually.

In Brazil, the Hospital das Clínicas in Sao Paulo conducted a study with 312 patients in 2010, showing that 23.5% of respondents did not understand well what they read. Of these, 60% had up to 7 years of study and 14% had education level between 8 and 11 years of study. Though a limited sample, represents a modern functional illiteracy, whose reality is seen worldwide not just with foreigners, but even with native speakers.

Many professionals like to use a technical language daily, and are sometimes derided by their colleagues when they are too clear with patients, or even reprimanded by professors in medical schools when do not use technical language knowledge. However, the overly technical language creates a barrier between the practitioner and the patient, one imagines that transmitted the information and the other tries to decipher what was said. Normally, after seeking clarification two or three times the patient feels embarrassed to question what is being said. Sometimes the practitioner try to explain again and again, but always using technical terminology not contributing to the prior explanation and still expressing anxiety as the patient and family seems to be suspicious or do not trust in its technical capacity.

Is up to the professional to identify the need of understanding or the level of literacy of the patient, even if he tries hard not to show his difficulty, this task is part of the professional role during the initial evaluation. To ask the patient if he/she understood the information or orientation transmitted usually leads to a positive response because many shall fear of pass themselves as illiterate or ignorant. There are very efficient techniques to evaluate the level of understanding that can be used as the known "teach back" process, asking to the patient to demonstrate or to explain in their own words what was told or taught. It is an action that takes time, but is highly effective to ensure that mistakes and failures do not occur in the future.

One should not assume that the patient actually understood everything that was said, not everyone has the ability to read well, understand and appropriately use medical terminology, even if considered simple. Although more common in the simplest social classes, this type of problem can occur at any age, race, social status or education.

An American organization AskMe3™ aimed to reduce errors and costs due to the low effectiveness of communication between patients and healthcare professionals, they noticed that people who have a low level of understanding of the terminology used in health, have the following problems.

• Are less likely to cooperate with the prescribed treatment when they are at their own care;
• Do not seek preventive care, more than doubling the risk of hospitalization;
• They are hospitalized about two days longer than adults with the same or greater degree of understanding;
• They need extra care that result in an additional cost to the health system, and can be up to four times more costly than a person with greater understanding.

Despite a study showing that the system had disappointing findings with patients participating in the AskMe3™ program published by the Annals of Family Medicine (8:151-159/2010), the problems cited above by the organization are real. Others have criticized the methodology of teach back in a parrot-like way, neglecting the importance to assure if the patient really understood the message, but criticism will always exist and there is no perfect system to get worldwide agreement without questions or without problems.

Among the public of health institutions many can use devices and special equipment such as crutches, wheelchairs and artificial limbs while others use hearing aids or otherwise that make its life easier every day. It is not uncommon the loss of these items while in hospital, the institution should provide the care needed when using regular devices mainly those necessary to have an effective communication while hospitalized.

Since the early stage of the care the staff must also inform the patient their rights, including the right to accept or refuse certain medical treatment. At any time of the treatment the staff can check where and when the patient needs more assistance and how it can affect the treatment, communicating the need to the rest of the team.

Finally, the time of hospitalization does not need to be traumatic and can be relieved with the introduction of complementary and differentiated services when noticed by the practitioner. Although it is not the primary purpose of the hospitalization, the treatment will have a new perspective with special attention from the hospitality team and making the stay as comfortable as possible. There are institutions that make the stay even more enjoyable, or at least not so bad, by offering menus with different dishes making the meal a pleasurable moment, offering extras such as fruits, amenities such as personal hygiene sets of famous brands, sandals, pajamas, among other items.

Evaluating the patient

After identifying the needs of the patient in the initial assessment, they must be registered in the medical records as soon as possible, in some accredited hospitals there is a period of time it needs to occur. The completeness and correctness of the medical records is a guarantee not only for the patient but also for the institution and the healthcare professionals themselves. The institution must also create, if does not exist, mechanisms to ensure that all members of the care team are aware of the patient's condition stated in the medical records.

A study of Fiocruz (Oswaldo Cruz Foundation) in Brazil analyzed the medical records of 750 patients in five hospitals in the city of Recife (PE) and found that about 60% of the records were incomplete, illegible or blank. From the hospitals evaluated, two were public, one private and two philanthropic. The issues analyzed ranged from very simple to indispensable information:

1. Basic data of the patient as the name and address
2. History of the disease including early symptoms, evolution and diagnosis

3. Main complaint and duration, if the disease was chronic or acute

4. Physical examination with details of the procedures performed

5. Personal and/or family historic of health problems

6. Diagnostic hypotheses

From the above, findings were classified as "bad" 59.9% of the medical records in the charity hospitals, 60% in the public hospitals and 68.5% in the private hospital. The effects of the problems arising from these failures may involve unnecessary costs with new tests, errors in medication administration, unnecessary procedures or misleading intervention, because the doctor or team responsible for an emergency care will not have the relevant information to decide what conduct to adopt during a critical moment. In case of malpractice suits, it can invalidate the main instrument for defending the professional and the institution. Although this is a sample in a single city, the reality does not seem to be different in many countries to a greater or lesser degree.

To guarantee the effective assistance during the patient evaluation is of paramount importance to identify and address the communication needs of the patient and establish an effective method of communication on special needs, such as:

• Use written methods (paper and pen)

• Use lip reading

• Use of sign language

• Use of a translator or interpreter

• Need for hearing devices

• Use of glasses or other equipment for improved vision

• Family support

• Use of electronic unit or voice equipment

• Other methods, verbal and nonverbal

Although widely known, is not always given due attention to crucial factors in the patient care due to problems as the short time given to every client and a proper medical records reading by the rest of the team. Every patient evaluation should be preceded by a brief introduction to the activities to be performed, establishing an effective relationship between the practitioner and the patient. Paying the due attention is possible to identify discrete and not always obvious barriers that affect the entire service, including:

• Foreign Patient

• Low level of awareness

• Illiteracy, functional illiteracy or difficulty of understanding

• Hostility with the staff

• History of stroke

• History of depression

• Agitation, confusion or delirium

• Patient intubated

• Patient sedated

• Contact after surgical procedures

• Patient alone or unaccompanied by family

• Visually impaired

• Hearing impaired and others that may exist

Despite the common affirmation from many health care professionals and institutions adds about the holistic treatment of the patient, and despite the best intentions the western medicine is fragmented and cartesian making difficult its practice. Requires attention to several factors inherent to the hospital care that need to be observed or not neglected for the most appropriate care, from the beginning to the end of care, such as:

• To help the patient to understand and to act using the information for their own benefit and as a valuable tool that increases the security within the hospital environment;

• To identify and to inform the rest of the team the needs for mobility of the patient if any;

• To identify the cultural bias, beliefs and religious practices of the patient that may influence part or all care received;

• To assess the needs, dietary restrictions and/or religious aspects that may influence the patient dietary during the hospitalization;

• Always ask the patient to indicate a person responsible for taking medical decisions and not just the person legally shown during the administrative procedure of admission;

• Always communicate the patient's needs to the medical and hospital staff who will take care of the patient. Of little value will hold all the information if not used properly;

• To address properly the communication needs of the patient during treatment;

• To monitor changes in the patient's communication profile. If any problem occur during the treatment, the patient will demonstrate through their mood, non-adherence to the treatment, interest for moving to another institution sometimes in a subliminal manner;

• To involve the patient and their families in the healing process, has been an indispensable tool for a better adherence to the treatment;

• Shape the written informed consent form for the patient's needs, taking into account that the existing form in most hospitals is ready and does not allow changes, or making changes or adjustments according to the needs of the patient;

• To educate the patient according to their needs, because most of the problems that occur is due to the fact that the patients were unaware of how the treatment is performed and what the practitioners want from him;

• Be sensitive to the cultural, religious, spiritual practices and beliefs of patients and its families. Some hospitals are unsuccessful to give attention to the religious needs of the patient;

Usually the family is included in the process of discharge and/or transfer of the patient, but no care is usually given to make sure everything went as planned, also known as the continuity of care. Besides checking what happened latter works like a barometer for future discharges or transfers ensuring the continuity of care at home or in the institution who receives the patient.

Chapter 3

HUMANIZING THE HOSPITAL CARE

Currently the world is becoming increasingly globalized with greater emphasis on technology, that has been maximized and sometimes raised to the level of panacea for solving the problems and almost all human ills. Optimistic projections are been made based on forecasts of new equipment and systems capable of the unthinkable for the benefit of the humanity and for future generations.

The unquestionable truth is that the technology has produced results and created benefits previously unimagined, promising a good future prospect for everybody. Now there is an increasing range of diseases and health problems that can be detected early, like cancer, making possible the cure, which was impossible without the technological advances in the diagnostic equipment industry.

The increase in the use of technology and the modernization of hospitals structure created a gap between the doctor and his patient. High investments in technology do not always mean improvement in the relationship with the patients, although it is of unarguable importance the early detection of diseases or the generation of new equipments with more accurate diagnoses.

Often, the tests only confirm what the doctor knows or serves to protect him in case of any future lawsuit. High-tech medical equipment are capable of high complexity tests, but are still used primarily for the same routine tests, and most professionals do not even know yet, what to do with the many possibilities the new equipment's are capable to do, like advanced results.

On the one hand we have the technological advances helping to prevent diseases and contributing for a longer and qualitative life. On the other we have a widening gap among many healthcare professionals, especially physicians and patients, creating a gap filled many times by a cold and inhuman medical equipment. Although the constant innovation and new technologies are necessary for the benefit of the humanity, the focus on humanizing health care institutions should not change with time. The patient is still the most important actor in the hospital theater, making the entire structure and human support exists only to mitigate and eliminate his pain and illness.

The patient is the reason for the existence of all health care institutions, so the patient is still more important than those often seen in hospitals as the great saviors or responsible for the healing and recovery of their health. Unlike the system that prevails in hospitals, the healthcare client is the most important person and who should converge all attention of the institution, contrary to the vision focused on physicians as modern gods. This is not to devalue the role of these recognized professionals, instead of it is to insert them in the real context and importance of their role in health institutions.

From the moment the patient is noticed about a required surgery followed by the hospital hospitalization, there are many questions not always answered in the first meeting. The time can bring others fears or inner fears of difficult externalization and some remain hidden for fear that these people may interpret it as weakness or cowardice. It is not easy to understand when we're across the table and in front of the patient, when the feeling of vulnerability and emotional instability is controlled by the patient who tries most often to mask or to make they appear stronger than actually is.

The moment of leaving the body and soul in others hands is extremely difficult for an autonomous and self-sufficient person. Suddenly a person will be

> **We can finally die in peace again!**
>
> "The development of technology cannot and should not distort the real medical mission: fighting diseases, prolonging life and ensuring a minimum quality, as well as to interact strongly with those who depend on our care, even when they are no longer curative. One must keep in mind that caring for dying is not at all, less important or worthy than caring to save. We cannot judge ourselves omnipotent gods, because, as such, we can enforce additional suffering to our patients and families, while trying to keep the "life" at all costs, especially when the death has already occurred: that, yes, a true medical error!"
>
> MD. Janice C. Nazareth

seen, touched and sometimes have his body invaded by equipments; even knowing that is performed by responsible and reliable professionals, it is not easy. These are moments of loss of control over himself, complete vulnerability and dependence. These are actions entrusted to technicians when undergoing major surgical treatments, that can be prolonged or be painful, not just for the body, but also for the mind of many people. How many men would like to tell what feels when evaluated by a proctologist? Or women telling the feelings about their treatment with an urologist?

When a healthcare professional becomes a patient and go through the same situation as the other patients, he feels the uncertainties and understands the anguish caused by an unnecessary and lengthy wait for the result of an examination or a medical report. They begin to note how much the empathy and clear and accurate information are important to those who are afflicted. Some even change significantly their relationship with their own patients, as demonstrated by doctors like Dr. Geoffrey Kurland in the book "My own medicine: the doctor's life as a patient", who candidly describe their fears, uncertainties and insecurities during the period in which he attempted to find out his disease and then to find the most appropriate treatment.

If the technology modernizes the hospital environment, on the other hand increases the distance between the doctor and the patient and making the healing process too cold. With currently problems related to abuses or sexual harassment the human contact, the physical examination and touching becomes increasingly hard and fast when it occurs. The human touch has

On a beautiful Saturday night came to the reception of a large hospital a young woman dressed as a bride and her husband, recently married and coming out of the church directly to the hospital before heading to the party with the guests. As the grandmother was hospitalized in the ICU could not attend the wedding and accomplish the dream of seeing her granddaughter she raised to marry.

Before the ceremony the couple had got a grandmother doctor's authorization to a brief visit to her after the ceremony, so the grandmother could see her in the wedding dress, as she always had dreamed. The bride had promised to visit her after her marriage, the patient was conscious and stable with no risk or severity in the context of her health.

However, the head of ICU, known for its rigidity, knew nothing about it and found an absurd a bride and groom wish to enter into an ICU at 10pm, although in a very special occasion. Despite repeated requests, attempts to speak with the doctor's patient who gave the authorization and a profusion of tears, the couple went to the reception party without the long awaited visit.

At the hospital they had not found the authorization nor were the ICU head doctor flexible enough to realize the importance of that moment in the life of those people. The next day while visiting her grandmother the granddaughter broke into tears in each other's arms. There are moments that can never be replaced and situations that will never be repaired. Like that in the earlier night.

decreased and often brings the message that the patient is someone to be avoided.

Large hospital complexes have signed expensive contracts with suppliers of technology, acquiring the latest equipment having the cutting edge technology. Again, they are increasingly necessary and useful to our modern medicine, but the managers most of time overlooks the most important part of the process, the human being, the patient on one side and the human capital on other, the most important asset of a hospital. It has been increasingly common the death in the midst of cold devices, cables and wires than in the comforting presence of a dear loved one, the so-called humanized death.

Not always the investment in technology are followed by investment in the skills and in the professionals, that can significantly improve the quality of care. The service in the health institutions has becoming increasingly cold, impersonal and based on protocols. The administrative workload and amount of work imposed on health professionals, puts the patient in a secondary position in the daily work routine. It is common in big hospitals to come and see some employees busied with internal administrative tasks, which at times cause the impression that the patient is bothering the professional to do their job.

This process seems to be increasingly common due to the requirements for filing reports, charts, forms with detailed data and other documents for internal control, to the health insurers and for government agencies. It reduces the time to care for patients showing the gap between the professional and the patient often against their will. The distance many managers keep from the front line prevents them from realizing these failures or loses the opportunity to rethink new processes from the point of view of the patient.

The patient point of view

The health and the life are the most precious assets the human being have, and when it is at stake emotional reactions are unpredictable. It is very common for patients and/or families under intense stress lose their mind and curse or use violence against some employees or the physician. Although it is not justifiable at any time, such action is the result of a person's despair mainly when there is a child involved or when something seems to go wrong. At such times, the patient or his family is not against the employees, but just for themselves.

What the patient sees when a surgery is needed is quite different from health care professionals who knows the hospital environment. At this time the hospitality services and the additional care provided in health institutions become an important part of the treatment, helping the patient to understand

and accept the new reality. The staff cannot avoid to involve or show indifference to the others suffering. It is time that the vulnerability of the human being has reached its critical point going beyond its control when showing the hidden emotions.

The hospital perceived image by the general public is formed in part by information gathered in the media, from third party or when someone use the service. Given the nature of the health care service whose consumption usually occurs in rare moments of a person life, the image of the institution is formed more by testimonials than a personal experience. Usually the media and testimonials focus the extremes, traumatic moments and great services done. These are critical moments that define the image that the patient can bear with them from the health institution. At times the least sensitive issue may pose a difficult barrier between the hospital and its client. This is why managers should pay more attention to their front line staff, giving them a better support to make them be supportive to the hospital clients.

When is the health or the life that is at stake, a person usually does not try to save or restrain to spend their money, in many cases, clear its financial resources or savings to ensure the best care. So, when a patient goes to a surgery the patient would not like to know that the professionals in charge had a bad night's sleep or are with family problems, because they know that this can affect the quality of the surgery results. Much less he wants to know that this surgery is the first of the doctor alone.

Everyone try to have the best within the limitations and possibilities of each one. In this moment the patient becomes keen to issues sometimes unnoticed by health care professionals. A sense of danger (also called the sixth sense) or an inner alert can make the patient aware of details that will influence his recovery such as comments, jokes, gestures and dubious or laughable words, minimizing the confidence that is placed in the institution. We all know that the communication becomes an important factor in the patient recovery, mainly when he feels unsafe. On the other hand, the same patient can see individual or collective efforts to guarantee his recovery.

Although the human factor will be the focal point for the patient care, the supporting infrastructure with additional patient services will bring a visibly differentiation of care. These additional services will help in two ways:

1 – Give direct support for the patient, providing him with comfort and well-being,
2 – Give support for the healthcare professionals to perform better their job.

Humanization comes from "the action to humanize", i.e.,

make human the act, the care or the medical attention. While some hospitals spends fortunes on new technologies, little sign has been shown that, equally or even more important than the technology itself is the human being, especially with the professionals who produces the main result the patient is looking for. Human experiences are successful or unsuccessful testifying favorably or negatively about the hospital, so hospital managers must choose what kind of hospital they want do deliver to their clients.

The approach about the quality in hospitals is a difficult task due to the different kind of services provided, and services are intangible assets perceived differently by each person. In health services we could say it is linked to healing or the cure. Despite all courses and training, the result is maybe dependent of environmental and human controlled and non-controlled factors.

It is possible to assure the right surgery in the right patient, to give the right medication to the right patient. However, there are subjective situations and critical moments as the death of someone that a few staff know how to deal with. Some people trying to help, in fact hurts the feelings or religion of the family. Normally there is no institutional policy to prepare the staff for such events, as the death, even for the best psychologists. Nowadays, not only the physician maintains contact with the family after the death of a patient, as other employees will continue the administrative services and support, most often without the due training.

More yet, usually those employees who are not well cannot deliver a good service. Workers also have financial problems, are victimized by illness, can have some family ill at home affecting productivity and the quality of attention. The way someone treat their customers is sometimes closely linked to his state of mind or to some physical dysfunction. Fatigue, stress, physical and mental dysfunction can reduce the quality of service rendered favoring problems and frictions among the staff. Rested and happy people tend to cope better with problems and aggressive behaviors revealed by third parties or clients.

Among the characteristics of health care facilities that could alleviate this situation or the stress of the job, is the lack of leisure and recreation spaces inside hospitals, where employees can relax during their leisure time with recreational activities by improving his mood and willingness to work. A lounge, a cozy space and small gym may seem absurd in a highly stressful environment such as hospitals, but are already used successfully in companies with fewer tendencies to tension in the human relations as banks, software and communication companies. The same could be done in hospitals with the aim to produce happier and rested professionals, affecting positively the way they treat the patients, caregivers, families and visitors.

Differentiating the humanization

Many health care professionals imagine that the humanization process is only human, need face to face contact, are embedded with empathy etc. when dealing with the client. However, this may surprise some professionals, but humanization can also be technical or mechanical and not just human. That is why engineers, architects and even financial managers can work with the humanization process within their area of expertise.

We can differentiate humanization in two ways

Criterion	Differences
Technical	Comprises technical and structural changes using protocols, technology and pre-determined concepts.
Human Relations	Comprises human actions and personal relationships based on empathy, attention and respect for the time of the patient and their family members.

Technically an hospital automatic bed with four engines contributes more to the humanization of care, rather than a mechanical bed that needs somebody's to help to change the position of the patient. The first grants autonomy, independence and a greater measure of comfort to the patient that can change its position when desired. The second will keep the dependency of a person whose constant requests for change of position will be stressful for the patient and his caregiver. It may seem simple and logical, but not all hospitals even in the richest countries have automatic beds everywhere.

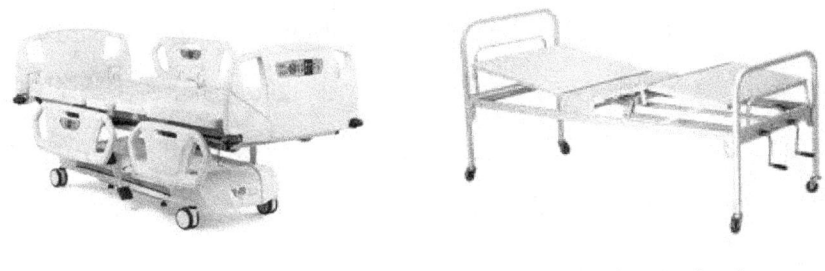

Automatic bed   Mechanic bed

The issue is not exactly the bed, but all the technical changes that a hospital can have to humanize the relationship between healthcare professionals and patients. The contact between the care team and physicians with the patient occurs daily in a fraction of the time the patient remains hospitalized, so it is obvious that more attention must be given to equipment's and services which will occupy the rest of the patient day. To leave the patient staring at the ceiling or to a bad television programming can lead him to think more of their disease than in health, and increases the chances of complaints by the attention given to the rare human contact in the hospital.

Thus, there is need to focus on technical changes to humanize the patient-hospital relation increasing the patient satisfaction, even with items related to accessibility using lifts and ramps uniquely for patients, visual and sound signals in accordance with the laws of each country, and especially the food. Instead of focusing on what the patient cannot eat, nutritionists and physicians can specialize in nutrition focusing in what the patient want to eat. In Sao Paulo, Brazil, some hospitals won gastronomy prizes with beautiful and tasty dishes, something unusual some decades ago. There is a change of mentality regarding hospital food, making them tasty and with a visual appeal to adults and children.

Although many hospitals want to customize the attention given to their patients, in practice is expensive to have a team that can give all the attention the patients needs. Many of the problems are related to emotional causes and require much time to minimize or solve the distress. Concierges and hospitality teams exist in many hospitals to meet the needs and demands of patients like hotels, but they sometimes may not meet the requests that are not practical or technical, as depression or people mentally ill who needs specific professional attention. Even for the hospital managers, the investment in a team composed of many employees cannot be justified with the care of a few at the expenses of others thousands of clients. It is increasingly common the quantitative model "**A**" of hospitality management outweigh the qualitative model "**B**" shown in this book.

Currently the trend is the increasing distance between health care professionals and the patients with a consequent reduction in the humanization process when based on personal relations practice and increased humanization technology. The humanization of health care services will go through a period where technical advances will reduce the pain and suffering of the patient with less invasive procedures or surgeries with smaller incisions, with the use of robots and the introduction of new equipments. The use of protocols and routines, that are valid and necessary, has becoming mechanical the personal relationships, distancing the most important agents in a hospital - the doctor and the patient.

Models: Quantitative X Qualitative

Model	The hospitality team results – Month: January
A	5786 patients visited. 3752 received praises and hospital compliments. 73.5% drop in complaints about the daily service in the rooms. 97% of patients felt important to receive the visit and wish to return to the hospital if needed. Detected and solved 181 cases that could generate public complaints or Lawsuits against the hospital.
B	186 patients visited, 72 were find with anxiety. 11 patients depressed or with ideas of suicide.

This widespread distance makes human relations increasingly less important, as seen in the clinics where the doctors can assess whether the patient is doing well or bad only through computerized tests. We can see reduced the former personal contact that existed with a good clinical evaluation of the patient, where the doctor could find common diseases only by signs such as swelling, skin color, physical evidence, etc. It does not mean that medicine has become less effective, unlike became more efficient, but more inhuman.

In the future probably there will be a return to the older model of customized human attention where each patient is unique, with lengthy consultations where the doctor hear and understand the whole patient, not just the disease. This will be a major differential in humanization of hospitals. But for this, two aspects of human relationships need to be reconsidered:

❖ It is harder to be more human than to be indifferent. And not everyone is willing to be more human in their professional relationships, choosing to ignore situations that do not interest him/her. No one wants to be ignored, but maybe is ignoring others when working.

❖ Everyone wants to be treated humanely, but not everyone is willing to treat others in the same way. Many people is seeking for the perfect human care as they seek some medical attention and hospital care, but not everyone is interested in making his/her care the best and more human when possible. I want a better care, but am I able to deliver this care at the same standard?

Stages of humanized care in the world

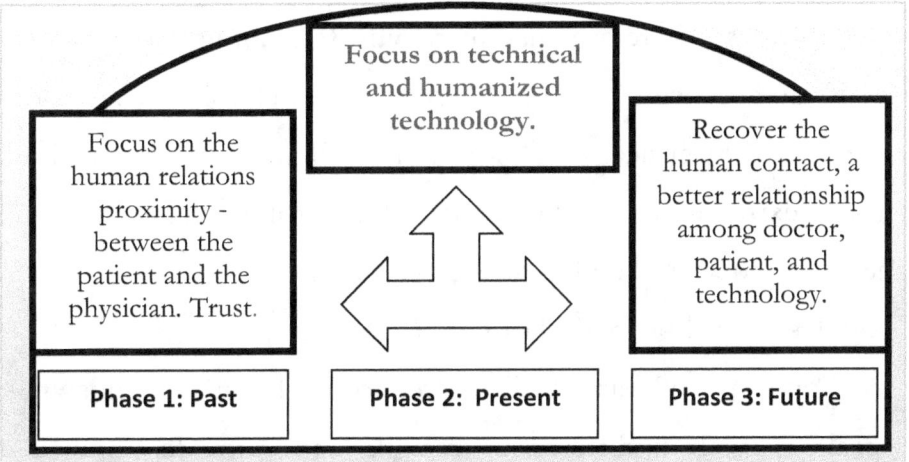

Focus on the human relations proximity - between the patient and the physician. Trust.	Focus on technical and humanized technology.	Recover the human contact, a better relationship among doctor, patient, and technology.
Phase 1: Past	**Phase 2: Present**	**Phase 3: Future**

When the patient is the problem

Although it has been coined the expression stating that the customer is always right, everyone knows that this is not an unquestionable truth, especially at hospitals. It's not difficult to see clients shouting angrily, complaining or crying loudly in hospitals, especially in emergency rooms. The first impression is that someone died, some injustice has been committed, there was a mistake or the patient and his family are being subjected to some arbitrary action.

The moment of care is a critical moment, with risks and difficulties involved ignored by some, and unnoticed by others. As strange as it may appear, there are patients who come to the emergency room of a hospital with interests that go beyond the medical care. There are customers who feel nothing and have to justify an absence from work or school, as well as there are those who arrive in critical condition and in some cases almost dead. These extremes make the work difficult for professionals who need to understand and treat everyone at the best way possible, in minutes or in short period of time.

Some people are really hard to deal with at hospitals, speaking with indifference, refusing to provide important information about health or personal habits or even mistreating the professionals doing their job. Often do so with arrogance and disrespect for the work of these professionals, but when a fault occurs in a hospital they present himself before the authorities humbly, as vulnerable and powerless victims during the treatment. Part of the problem lies with the institutions themselves with its policy of "no confrontation" letting the situation remains unpunished. For employees offended is the fear of acting alone and being laid off or suffer other kinds of moral violence, beyond those already submitted in advance by the patient and their families.

As absurd as it seems, is more common than someone think employees to be mistreated by patients, especially in private hospitals. Although it is not so evident, when attacks occurs or there are problems that cannot be clearly proven by the employee, the law tends to favor the patient who is *a priori* in disadvantage, weakness and dependency of care. And there are patients who take advantage of their professional position as a authorities, police officers, politicians and even doctors. The offenses range

> A tall and strong man appearing little more than 50 years old, breaks into the Admission's late in the evening and in front of several clients in a loud voice threatens to put the hospital name on television and in newspapers for an inadmissible failure, what seemed to be no problem for him as a famous journalist known throughout the country.
>
> He accused the hospital to keep his wife in the hospital unnecessarily without any treatment, and after the complaint someone sent a fruit basket to minimize the situation. Other patients waiting at the same place have expressed concern finding the situation absurd.
>
> After listening patiently, the head of Admissions checked what happened and explained clearly. The patient refused to undergo a surgery until the arrival of her husband that night coming from another state, allowing only one tooth extraction that afternoon which could compromise their future cardiac functions. When there is a tooth extraction is usual to send a basket of fruits, juices and soft beverages to the patient, with the usual meal.
>
> Aware that her husband was nervous and afraid of his aggressive behavior, the fearful wife said nothing after his arrival, admitting only when she was questioned in front of her husband and the Concierge.
>
> The husband did not to apologize for the insults and threats made, and neither the patients and companions who witnessed the first scene knew the truth because they had already gone.

from irony, racist terms, humiliation and even mild attacks, most without any means of evidence or witnesses. At such times, it is up to the professional to act responsibly and do not hesitate to look for their rights, especially recording the moment when such situations occurs, without compromising the privacy.

Not everyone looking for a hospital are actually seeking treatment, the medical refusal to give what the patient wants may result in complaints, threats and even attacks. Some expected that the doctor can simply guess the problem he/she has, or think they are waiting for too long for test results, as if they were ready in a minute or so. Some people complain for being admitted in a hospital and others complain of not being admitted. In some cases, the lack of insurance coverage or the need to carry out some expensive procedure leads family members to unnecessary friction with the staff who serve them, who is just trying to help them.

Part of the problem is related to the expectation of the patient and his family members, when they are not satisfied it becomes a complaint embodied in the first person, they think is creating an obstacle or when the staff give a negative answer. For many people, the health care institutions should work according to "their" own way, and any other proceeding necessary to ensure patient safety is seen as unnecessary bureaucracy. However, when problems occurs, usually these same people are those who claim that the correct procedures adopted by the institution were not followed properly. Among them are those protocols used in hospitals, some of which are repeated with the aim to increase safety and reduce errors and failures, how to check the name and procedure to be performed at different times of service.

All hospital staff usually strives to make possible to all patients and families meet their expectations, but difficult situations and misfortune can always occur causing a false impression to them that the service is bad. The goal should be always provide the best care regardless of the client and the situation experienced. Hospital managers need to prepare the staff to deal with critical situations, continually training them and supporting them through psychological support and creating mechanisms to help them to relieve tensions. Who treats and helps people, sometimes also needs help to keep doing a good job.

Managing the patient-hospital relationship

As usually happens in all kinds of business relationship, not always the health client-hospital relationship is healthy all the time, and some situation may cause dissatisfaction, can leave patients discontent and even result in lawsuits, although the rule observed is normally "satisfaction". When the problem is with the doctor, there are fewer complaints from those people afraid of retaliation or loss of quality in the service. That's why many customers prefer to look for another hospital and another doctor.

Although the hospital is the kind of business that is unlikely to have lack of customers, the business can face a noticeable reduction in the amount of the preferred customers, and attracting new quality customers are expensive. Usually the patient looks for a doctor, this is what professionals say that physicians have patients not hospitals. If the doctor goes away, the richest patients usually go together.

Clients and families are increasingly aware of their health problems, rights and options existing in the market. It is not uncommon claims at professional bodies such as boards of medicine and the justice to repair damages or grant rights, or lawsuits against insurers, medical health plans or hospitals. To pay attention to the client relationship and the quality of hospital care provided can reduce the dissatisfaction and lawsuits, making the patient a source of revenue and not a headache.

The existence of good ears in departments such as the Customer Service, allows patients and their families to feel safe and supported upon the occurrence of some internal problem or doubtful situation. Some cultures have a bad preconceived image of one who complains about any care or service, resulting in the patient preferring to look for another hospital to have to face a slow and exhausting process to have their problems solved. In practice there is a drain of precious resources for other institutions that offer similar or better quality services even at a higher cost.

In developing countries there is still the divine role of the physician, being considered absolute and unquestionable truth their verdicts. They don't delegate to the patient the right to decide what treatment he wants to follow or presenting the treatment tailored to their convictions and not necessarily considering the patient choice. The treatment ends up being imposed without considering other possibilities (Mezomo, 1995).

Also, when family members look for a doctor for more information they are often received with dislike, getting answers in a hurry, evasive, with technical terminology or imprecise information. This situation happens even in highly developed countries like USA and England. Maybe, they are not bad professionals, maybe because some doctors cannot give the luxury of dispensing more than a few scarce minutes to their patients, due to strenuous routines and jobs in different hospitals. It is not the patient problem and need to be fixed by the hospital.

At times of sadness and pain every word of a doctor may be misunderstood and give rise to various interpretations by the relatives of a patient in critical condition. The physician and writer Moacyr Scliar wrote: *"Every word spoken by a doctor to his patient is a verdict. As the writer, he should consider every word and know how to use it with extreme rigor."* Another factor of great importance is the treatment and care of the soul, the spirit and not only the body, the physical appearance. As Buchalla (2004) cites addressing the humanization of care in hospitals, "... *the lack of technology and resources are offset by long and affectionate conversations. Sometimes that's all the patient needs."*

While we notice an increase in the technology used in hospitals we also realize an increased in the distance between doctor and patient. The valuable human relations have been reduced each day instead of growing, especially when the trust between the patient and the hospital should be maximized before a surgery that may result in death. The high investments in technology and medical equipment does not always means improvement in diagnostic results or the accuracy of them. This information is currently undervalued even by those who believe in the history that the more modern the hospital, the more reliable it is.

To understand the differences, the health care costs or treatments in the United States are on average 60% higher than the Canadian model and 100% higher than the European model. Each model has its specific features, rather than to say that an American model is better than the European or Canadian. To possess the most modern medical equipment is also not a guarantee of better results. The diagnostic accuracy was studied in Germany involving the years 1958, 1968, 1978 and 1988, resulting in the evaluation that the use of technology did not improve the diagnosis given by the doctors. We still have to remember the absence of advanced equipment such as MRI or ultrasound and other in these decades. The physician ability is still the best resource in a hospital.

Meyer (2002) addresses the technical medicine and the new therapeutic methods adopted in recent years, which may deviate the doctor from the more human medical procedures and their own ability to care for their customers.

> *To regain their full responsibility, the physician must learn to measure the capacity of the means available to him than those from their predecessors: a weighted appreciation of the nature of progress is essential to the perception of its advantages and its dangers. To preserve the humanity of medicine, there must be a reflection on the respect of human personality that can be compromised by new therapeutic approaches, those usable before birth and before death.*

Often the tests or their results are only required to justify what the doctor already knows, even to compensate his lack of experience or expertise, to protect themselves in case of any lawsuit (defensive medicine), or to support the diagnosis and prognosis in situations involving medical doubts. There is no question here about the need of exams and the undeniable importance of the new technology in which they have become indispensable, but about the space they took over in our modern medicine replacing the expertise of the physician. The perception of the doctor and his ability to penetrate the human soul to uncover the problems that affect the body resulting in diseases, have not yet been supplanted by any equipment. Here, perhaps, one of the most beautiful and divine gifts that a physician can have.

There are many humanized and competent medical professionals who work in hospitals spending their life to treat patients, even when they are unpaid or did not receive what they deserve for their hard work and heroic conduct. Some of them works in undignified conditions in hospitals that do not provide a good structure and decent support, while others devote part of their little free time to care for those in need in nongovernmental organizations. However, it is necessary to rethink about the divine role and "unwritten" rule that the doctors are almost worshiped by in many places. The State University of São Paulo (UNESP) conducted a study that showed a revealing snapshot of the doctors at that time. According to the study:

Percentage of doctors	Medical findings of the study
73%	Recognize that have prescribed medicines without knowing the exact composition of these drugs.
71%	Forget to warn the patient about the reactions (side-effects) caused by the use of two or more drugs.
72%	Said that works in two or more hospitals, which prevents them to continue studying.
62,5%	Do not attend medical conferences/congress.
40%	Do not read medical journals or scientific publications.

Source: Unesp/2004

Managers and physicians should be aware of their own needs to analyze the resources they have to invest in the essential, not overlooking the human side as less important. Some valuable strategies see beyond the premises focusing too in the treatment of the body and soul of the patient. There is a need for more action and less discussion among the society, health care administrators and especially the government when involving the human most important asset, it's health, it's life. There is plenty of room for change to better, to bring back the trustful relationship among healthcare professionals and patients looking for medical care. As written by Dr. Philippe Meyer:

A time to look, to exchange a word or a gesture cannot be measured, the quality of the presence is for the patient an invaluable asset, and to the doctor should be a source of satisfaction. The image of a physician cannot be elusive, impenetrable or absent. The requirements of technical, administrative or economic obligations should never forget this duty of humanity to one that delivers itself confident.

Complementary Therapies

The practice of medicine is characterized by the treatment of symptoms and diseases, known as allopathic medicine or the medicine of the opposites. With increasing awareness about the importance of prevention, the medicine itself has become more holistic in contrast with the focus solely on the specialization, understanding how psychosocial factors influence the loss of harmony and internal balance triggering the mechanisms that lead to diseases. Some treatments are turning to the holistic side of the man with the use of not-so-conventional ways and not always widely accepted complementary therapies like the use of colors, food and smell within the hospital environment.

The importance of complementary actions to the medical treatment can help, for example, a patient with little appetite to have the taste stimulated by having a colorful food (chromotherapy), which exhale a pleasant odor (aromatherapy) and that is tasty (gastronomy). These are no medical treatments, but may contribute to the well being of the patient encouraging him to adhere to the treatment. This is why health care professionals must increasingly look to complementary treatments that has always been present in everyday life. They are invaluable tools to make the treatment experience or medical intervention less unpleasant, especially in hospitals.

Chromotherapy

The colors have always exerted a great influence on people's mood and behavior, been embedded in the cultural context of virtually all peoples around the world. From colors that indigenous people used in their body paintings to reflect the sympathy or readiness for war to the modern tones that enhance the sensuality of a female skin, we usually use the colors even in everyday talks. Occasionally we hear that a person was purple with rage, who smiled yellow (faint smile), that the economic situation is black. We drive our attention to the colors of traffic lights to move forward or to stop, and when we prepare the room for the a new baby, usually blue for boys and pink for girls. Not mandatory of course.

Color therapy (or chromotheraphy) has been considered by many experts as an effective way to establish or restore harmony and emotional, mental and physical balance through the use of colors in the environment or with the direct application in humans. It is undeniable that some colors can make people depressed as black and alerts or agitated as red. Within the hospital environment is even more important because the patient is vulnerable to the external influences affecting unconsciously emotionally and psychologically.

Given this finding, hospital architects and managers should pay attention to the use of colors in the staff clothing, hospital furniture, floors, walls and especially within the inpatient units by interfering in the routine and well-being not only of patients but also with the health professionals. The appropriate use of colors results in less emotional stress of patients and reduces the opaque colors that permeate the majority of hospitals environment. The colors can influence differently the human body causing irritation, restlessness, drowsiness influencing the behavior and acting as a natural sedative.

Administrative areas like the admissions can receive stronger and more vivid colors with bands, stripes or in parts of the wall in order to maintain the professionals alert and motivating visitors to stay less time on site. The lighting system should also be observed, leaving the environment brighter, although it should be in accordance with labor standards where necessary. Corridors and walkways can receive part of the strong colors in the walls or floors stimulating agility and keeping the senses sharp, and graphics on floors and walls that lead people unconsciously to waiting rooms and exits. In the open areas or waiting rooms the color must be a replicator of the sunshine keeping people awake, and lighting up the other areas of the building.

The patient apartments may use flat wooden panels to cover some walls and the medical equipment, keeping them visible only when in use by the staff. In addition to the usual colors used at hospitals, it is possible to use light blue and light green with different shades, colors that are calming. The aisles of the pediatric unit must receive bright colors with images of animals and toys when applied in the wall or in the floor in bold colors like red, yellow, blue and orange. Shades of yellow and light gray can also be applied to patient care rooms and the ceiling. Despite being present everywhere, white is a universal color that denotes purity, cleanliness and harmony useful in many different environments, preferably with the use of other highlighting color attracting the attention of the people eyes.

Colors can also be used in hospitals whose spaces are often cramped and make the place seems tight. For example, when the ceiling is lower than usual it can be painted with a lighter color than the walls to give the impression of elevation. To lower the ceiling, it is the reverse action painting the ceiling with a darker color than the walls. The white increases the feeling of space while black causes tightness. Some colors are used by therapists to reduce anxiety and distress, others to solve skin problems and as a natural tranquilizer in some places.

Obviously the colors of the room walls will not heal the patient within the hospital, however, contribute in making the stay more enjoyable affecting the state of mind during the treatment. Also, the slightly stronger colors used correctly in environments and in the appropriate extension to the spaces will not make the patients sicker or leaving the professionals fatigued.

The use of bright colors makes the hospital alive, less sad and less apathetic, affecting positively the patient's mood, also the visitors and keep professionals attention, especially in collective spaces with human constant interaction. Additionally fountains can be used in strategic locations, internally or in winter gardens with sculptures and green gardens, changing the cold and rigid hospital pattern and turning it in a warmer and friendly environment.

Aromatherapy

The use of scents, perfumes, oils and other extracts with pleasant odors have been used for millennia by the Greeks, Egyptians, Romans and Chinese people to treat patients or for the good mental and physical wellbeing. The use of aromatic oils have been widely applied in complementary therapies of Indian and Chinese cultures seeking to stimulate the sense of smell through the scent, inhalation of vapors or use of ointments and oils for massage due to their anti-inflammatory, analgesic, antiseptic and relaxing characteristics.

Some essences are presented in the form of gel, cream, ointment and oil that can be inhaled or used to massage parts of the body by reducing pain, as expectorants and used in baths causing a feeling of well being that affects the person's psychological state. One of the oldest drugs used in Brazilian households is made from menthol, camphor and eucalyptus oil been widely used for inhalation and chest and back massage relieving symptoms of flu and colds, also relieving chest and body aches.

The scents can be relaxing, stimulating, healing, aphrodisiac, tonic or take other action as being antidepressant. The most common essences are geranium, jasmine, lavender, sandalwood, fennel, orange blossom, bergamot, clove, peppermint, eucalyptus, rosemary, mint, pine, cinnamon, jasmine, rose, patchouli, eucalyptus, thyme, cypress among many others used in perfumes and cosmetics that are used daily mainly by women and children. The composition of certain plants and oils can generate new aromatic essences with different physical and psychological benefits.

The human sense can detect the scent of a washed cloths or the smell of a delicious meal prepared with care. The aroma associated with the colors and flavor of the food can produce pleasant sensations to the hospitalized patient. However there still is a great resistance among the physicians. The health care professionals needs to understand that the scents and perfumes are not intended to be used everywhere, or to replace any treatment but to cause positive feelings that will stimulate the patient to accept and contribute with the care provided in the hospitals.

Obviously there are allergic people that cannot inhale certain substances and shall avoid it, mainly inside the patient room and areas of admissions. But, it is unarguable that people prefer to stay in places exhaling nice fragrances, as waiting rooms and spaces used by the employees. The scents and perfumes can be used with discretion to be slightly noticed by everybody.

Music Therapy

Music therapy is the use of music and other sounds as a stimulus, helping the person recovery at many levels mental, social, and even used to physical rehabilitation of the person. It has been used in the rehabilitation of individuals with mental disorders, speech and hearing impairments, especially those who have suffered stroke and injuries that compromise any of the functions of sense. The use is very wide as to encourage learning and social integration due to its proper characteristics causing a relaxation and a better rapport between people.

It has long been known that music stimulates several functions of the brain being used successfully with children from an early age, to have a peaceful sleep or to stimulate the intellectual development of children and adolescents. Add to this the benefits that the music brings to peace, tranquility and happiness to hear songs that were part of one's life.

In the hospital environment it is no different and again it does not replace the medical treatment. The therapy can be used in a successful manner within hospitals aiding the treatment during the patient stay. Even when there is no medical indication, the music has a positive effect on mood and predisposition of the patient to accept medical intervention. Regardless of scientific studies, musical performances are always nice especially when they reach the patient at hospitals.

The hospital environment can and should be filled with pleasant music, resulting in touring musical performances by musicians inside hospitals, sometimes small concerts with many instruments and there is also hospitals with their own choir. Many doctors aware of the benefits of music have encouraged their patients to make best use of this resource as complementary therapy for many cases such as arthritis, Alzheimer's and other disorders.

When the music comes to the hospital it should mainly arrive firstly to the patient. Many hospitals in almost all continents have musical presentations performances in waiting rooms and entrance halls, benefiting patients while waiting or in transit, in addition to benefitting staff and visitors who stop to listen and be enchanted by the melodies of pianos, violins and other instruments.

What needs to occur with greater intensity is the music to reach the patient inside the hospital, because in most cases, he or she is far or does not participate in the presentations. Especially in prolonged hospital stay the patient has no contact with the outside world except through the television. Although is difficult the logistics of making the music accessible to hospitalized patients, those who can walk or be transported without major risks could participate in recitals and other performances, even if they occur in environments uniquely reserved to them.

The music becomes more than a hospital business card for all the people around, and should be used most to benefit the patient who should be the goal of the action and it's the biggest beneficiary. Maybe, all pianos at a hospital lobby can be used extensively some day and not just in special occasions.

Gastronomy (High Cuisine)

It's been for a long time that the meals in hospitals were only to supply the need of food for patients. The terminology more suitable to this change is "gastronomy" or "high cuisine" reflecting the preferences of patients, families and professionals within hospitals. In recent years nutritionists have realized the importance of a savory menu for the patients, a process initiated by the addition of "chefs" in some hospitals and later with the physicians approval after realizing that the diet also contributes indirectly to the improvement of the patient recovery.

Now is widely noticed that the food in hospitals can bring aromas, flavors and colors that stimulate the eyes, the smell and taste. It is possible to insert new ingredients that bring to the mind of the patient, his memory of taste and the taste of homemade food. With technology facilitating the distribution and maintenance of the flavor and the food heated while delivering to the patients, now customized menus that meet the most demanding palates is allowed everywhere.

Even in cases in which the food restriction is big, it is still possible to act with creativity in the presentation of the meals and the decoration of the dishes, mainly for children. Attention must also involve the crockery and cutlery used, which are part of the whole system involving good napkins and a nice service made preferentially by waiters. All professionals involved need to engage in the process, from the waitress or waiter who serves and collects the dishes noting some negative reaction from the patients to nutritionists who need to make daily visits to the patients to find their preferences and tailor the menu appropriately. To turn the need of food in a pleasant and tasty experience, surely contributes to the patient satisfaction and promote the image of the hospital in the market.

This is perhaps one of the most obvious mindset changes within the hospitals, with the inclusion of chefs and others specialists in nutrition to prepare differentiated meals working with physicians and healthcare professionals improving the patient's satisfaction. It's really interesting how in a few years, many health care professionals who have before disdained the appreciation of gastronomy inside the hospital environment, now discuss and write about the importance of patients feeding and the improvement of the institution's image through this actions.

Other therapies may be used in a successful manner, depending on the institution and the doctor. Usually what we see is the resistance to implementing such actions in major hospitals due to not direct scientific evidence of the benefits of some therapies that are compatible with the treatment, and also the logistics and the investment done by mobilizing several employees for the activity. Although recognized as beneficial it is not something essential within the hospital environment, some therapies have been of little used, with the exception of music therapy and the growing importance of the high cuisine in the hospitals. Maybe in the future with further studies, doctors and hospital managers can learn how such actions add value to the product "treatment" offered by hospitals.

Chapter 4
ERRORS AND FAILURES INSIDE HOSPITALS

Despite it is not something we like to talk about, this is an issue which should have further discussion and the growing involvement of health care institutions in the prevention of medical malpractice, nursing malpractice or other that results in damage to health or loss of life of the patient. Usually it comes to light and is debated by the population only when an error occurs or a grotesque death is reported in the media. According to the World Health Organization (WHO) in the annual survey of the patient (WHO - Patient Safety Research) for 2009 "Each year, tens of millions of patients worldwide suffer disabling injuries or death due to unsafe medical care. Almost one in ten patients is harmed while receiving care in a hospital well-financed and technologically advanced. "

Surgery in a wrong member, in a wrong patient, medication errors, failure of diagnosis or during treatment among other incidents occur with an intensity greater than that observed in the media as objects and materials left inside the patient during surgeries. But, what is an error? "Error can be defined as the failure of a planned action to be completed as intended (e.g. error

90

of execution) or the use of a wrong plan to achieve an aim (e.g. error of planning)[1].

And what can be considered a medical error? The medical error can be understood as a failure of the physician in the exercise of their activity and whose main features are the recklessness, negligence and malpractice. When using this expression, the first impression is that the doctor made a mistake that this is not necessarily the situation in all cases. It is also necessary to understand and differentiate the failure, and what occurs when a certain expectation is not met due to factors unrelated to the desire and interest of the physician and the care team. The problem can also be related to the others professionals involved in the action and not the physician.

In some countries there is less registered information about failures or medical errors or malpractice if compared to those errors committed and reported by nurses. The figures released are abysmally lower than the practice shows in the real life. The lawsuits in the justice help to assess people's awareness about their rights, but do not necessarily reflect the true picture of events in the country. From 2002 to 2008 the cases tripled in the Superior Court of Justice of Brazil, from just 120 to 398 in a country now with more than 210 million inhabitants (2018 data). Deficiencies in communication, lack of proper record in the

---

[1] *To Err Is Human: Building a Safer Health System. National Academy Press.*

medical records and sub-notification in reporting the incident contribute to the existing framework.

	What is it?
Recklessness	Occurs when the professional assumes certain risks for the patient during a procedure without having the scientific support for the procedure, acting rashly, unreasonable or without the necessary caution.
Malpractice	Occurs when a professional performs a certain procedure for which is not enabled, which has no theoretical preparation and/or practical due to inexperience, inability or ignorance.
Neglecting	Occurs when a professional acts with indolence, passivity or inaction and does not providing the necessary care to the patient, characterizing as an omission act.

There are several factors contributing for a healthcare professional error, for example, do not to follow protocols, the excessive hours of work common to medical and nursing staff in some countries, poor information; poor doctor-patient communication, doctor to doctor and nurse to doctor communication, few exams and poor or insufficient physician/nurse training to perform some procedures among other reasons. If the actual amount of failures and medical and nursing errors are not known in many countries, the data is a little more accurate in others as in the United States.

In the book "To Err is Human: Building a Safer Health System", Linda Kohn, Janet Corrigan, and Molla Donaldson from the IOM (Institute of Medicine) report estimates that between 44000 and 98000 people die in America each year due to healthcare professional errors. The malpractice in the country has cost more lives than the 43458 deaths in motor vehicle accidents, the 42297 deaths from breast cancer, and that 16516 deaths from HIV.

According to the book, over six thousand people die in America each year due to workplace injuries, while only deaths related to medical errors exceed seven thousands if happens in or out of the hospitals environment. The costs involving the loss of income, family members and unnecessary medical expenditures are estimated between US$ 17 and US$ 29 billion, more than half due to the cost of the extra care needed.

These data were obtained in two large studies carried out in the states of Colorado and Utah (Utah and Colorado Study), and the other in New York (Harvard Medical Practice Study), both in the United States. It's possible to see that the estimates have very different results (more than 100%)

It happened at hospitals

The known health care reporter for the Boston Globe, Betsy Lehman, died from an overdose during chemotherapy.

The patient Willie Kind had the wrong leg amputated.

Ben Kolb was eight years old when he died during "minor" surgery due to a drug mix-up.

Source: To Err is Human: Building a Safer Health System

between 44 thousands and 98 thousands deaths of preventable medical errors possibly due to temporal changes in the health system, evolution of health care and years used for each study group.

The group of Colorado and Utah used data from 1992, while the New York group used data from 1984. It is noticed that with increasing regulation, security systems and hospital accreditation there was a reduction in medical and medication errors occurred annually. It is noteworthy that there were 33.6 million admissions to U.S. hospitals during 1997. Each study presents the percentage of adverse events (AEs) reported as shown in the table below.

USA Research States	Adverse Events percent of hospitalizations	Adverse Events that lead to death	Preventable Adverse Events	Death due to medical error
Colorado/ Utah	2.9%	6.6%	53%	44000
Nova York	3.7%	13.6%	58%	98000

In the same book the authors cited a more recent study in two major American university hospitals, where two of every 100 admissions had some type of medication errors related to the patients. Only those adverse events increased hospital costs by about $ 4,700, occurring at the same rate would be $ 2.8 million annually to a hospital with 700 beds, and if applied throughout the country the avoidable costs would exceed $ 2 billion. In addition, approximately one in every 131 outpatient deaths and one of each 854 inpatient deaths is due to medication errors.

Many researchers have developed their work and published books and scientific articles showing how this problem is more common in hospitals than we think. Leape *et al.* (1993)[2] studied the types of errors that include the most common surgeries in the wrong member, adverse events of medication, errors during transfusions, patient falls among other events occurring within the hospital environment, classifying them as follows:

Diagnostic	Treatment
Error or delay in diagnosis, Failure to employ indicated tests, Use of outmoded tests or therapy, Failure to act on results of monitoring or testing.	Error in the performance of an operation, procedure or test, Error in administering the treatment, Error in the dose or method of using a drug, Avoidable delay in treatment or in respond to an abnormal test inappropriate (not indicated) care.
Preventive	Other
Failure to provide prophylactic treatment, Inadequate monitoring or follow up of treatment.	Failure of communication, Equipment failure, Other System failure.

In addition to adverse events (AE) that can occur in hospitals, there is also the so-called sentinel events (SE) that are

[2] Source: *Leape; Lucian; Lawthers; Ann G.; Brennan, Troyen A.; et al. Preventing Medical Injury. Qual. Rev. Bull. 19 (5) 144-149, 1993.*

unexpected occurrences with injuries, physical or psychological danger or even with the death of the patient. Sentinel events can be the unexpected or unexplained death of a patient, the surgery in the wrong site or wrong patient, medication errors, transfusion reaction, permanent loss of function, anesthetic events, adverse reactions to drugs, diagnostics, pre-and post-operative different from other.

> ### It happened in a hospital...
>
> Physician distracted during a surgery and operates the wrong knee of a 50 years old patient. The patient with an injured left knee meniscus was operated by mistake in his right knee. To make matters worse the wrong knee surgery had a thrombosis.

Usually in hospitals when an error occurs, the first reaction is to look for someone to be blamed, however, even in apparently simple situations which we see is a set of failures that contributed to the error occurrence. To find a guilty person will not solve the problem of the hospital or even the patient, though perhaps initially meets the wishes of the victim for justice that needs to realize that some action was taken. Health care institutions seem to have realized the importance of preventing errors and improving patient safety by developing processes and protocols that aim to prevent the conditions for the convergence of errors, eliminating them.

Although reported only when tragic cases occur stirring the society through the media, medical errors occur with a greater frequency than imagined by most people. It is not usually the technical inability or difficulties of students to access to quality schools, despite the proliferation of courses worldwide, health care professionals are among the most qualified of its countries. It is up to the managers or team medical chief or hospital CEO to assess whether any individual does not meet the expectations required by the function. Mostly what is seeing is a system failure or managing internal processes that lead to error, often noticeable in the earlier stages of patient care, cannot be attributed only to chance.

Looking to the activity from another perspective, is possible to understand the difficulties involved in the care of a sick patient. After arriving at the emergency department health care professionals need to identify the problem and present a solution as fast as possible. It is very simple when the action involves a vehicle repair, to replace a door or to stop a leak. Just unplug, disassemble, replace and rewire everything back to normal. If it still does not work, proceed to rework and correct any mistakes without major problems.

With humans the situation is quite different and so much more complex, there is no possibility to turn off the patient, much of the service occurs without both parties know yet what is wrong and there is no possibility for constant correction. In summary, there is no room for failure when they may incur in damage or death of the patient. However, doctors and other health care professionals are not gods. They are human with fears, feelings and liable to err like any other human being. These are people who mourn the loss and rejoice with the improvement and healing of a patient. Although it is unacceptable, human being can commit mistakes and errors despite their dedication and care. There are doctors who pride themselves on never having signed a death certificate, others who live with this reality every day. And it doesn't mean one is better prepared than the other.

Grounded in the Hippocratic principle of "*primum non nocere*" first do not cause any harm, a professional cannot exempt itself from blame and responsibility when he makes a mistake, or simply put the blame for a lapse or mistake in others. The errors are typically of execution when there is a failure of a planned action to be completed as planned, or of planning when there is the use of a wrong plan to achieve a goal. Thus, the process begins wrongly or some stage of the process is not fulfilled making possible the failure occurs. Among the reasons contributing to this practice in many countries are poor qualifying, many jobs or/and long working hours.

It happens many times with those with more than one job or that works in more than one hospital. Is well known in many countries like Brazil about nurses employed in two or three hospitals while doctors works in several. Many of them works 12 hours in a hospital, 6 or 12 hours at another hospital usually on night shifts and there are still those who attend a college with two jobs. Even if he/she lives near to the job there is no way one person perform their tasks accurately well or do not make any mistakes at some point in this routine. The result can be difficulty in concentration, attention to what they are doing, irritability, drowsiness or fatigue and other effects that may result in failures during patient care.

> ***Adverse Event*** (***AE***) are unwanted complications arising from patient care, not necessarily a natural progression of the patient's underlying disease.

Likewise, there are doctors who works in more than one hospital, also doing nights shifts, in emergency rooms and still works in his own clinics during the day. There is no way to maintain the same level of attention and understanding that they would if they were rested. It is no coincidence the increase in obesity and others unusual diseases in the medical profession and the increased stress with patient care. Although no one cannot directly attribute the errors in hospitals due to these factors. The lack of studies certainly contributes to its occurrence. In a survey conducted in Brazil with doctors who works in private hospitals (59%) and public (41%), some of them had up to six jobs. About 27% of the physicians have at least three jobs.

Number of Jobs	Percentage of physicians working
1	14%
2	34%
3	27%
4	15%
5	6%
6	4%

Awareness of the need to increase patient safety can be seen with the launch of the World Alliance for Patient Safety by the World Health Organization (WHO) in 2005. The WHO appointed the Joint Commission International (JCI) as a Collaborating Centre, non-governmental accreditation organization for quality processes to develop and disseminate the measures in order to encourage improvements in care provided to patients. There was created six international patient safety goals with an expected positive impact on the hospital routine, as observed in the table below.

Goal 1	Goal Requirements
Identify Patients Correctly	Failure in the correct identification of patients can result in serious errors such as surgery, drug administration and/or blood transfusion to wrong patients. The risk increases when the

| | patient is unconscious or unattended. |

Hospitals should use identification systems such as bracelets with name, date of birth, registration information as numbers, bar code, etc., Verbal and electronic systems check is also useful to ensure that the correct patient is receiving the care provided. The institution must use at least two means of identification of the patient.

Goal 2	Goal Requirements
Improve Effective Communication	Communication errors, incorrect or ambiguous interpretation can result in irreversible damage to the patient.

Hospitals should implement mechanisms such as "read back" to those who is receiving the information repeating the information conveyed, improved medical writing and use of electronic systems to ensure that the received message is the same broadcasted. Some countries does not permit verbal orders or orders made by telephone, while it is permitted in others.

Goal 3	Goal Requirements
Improve the Safety of High-alert Medications	Improving drug safety surveillance of electrolytes at high drug concentrations are considered of high risk, requiring greater security in preparing and administering to the patient. Are considered the potassium chloride, potassium phosphate, sodium chloride >0.9%, etc. The concentrated electrolytes need to be removed from patient care units.

Hospitals need to create security systems such as storage in safes, in pharmacies, restricted to handling only to nurses or pharmacists, electronic control output and red labels distinguishing them from others medicines.

Goal 4	Goal Requirements
Eliminate Wrong-site, Wrong-patient, Wrong-procedure Surgery	Ensure surgeries with correct local intervention, correct procedure and correct patient, through an effective communication between surgical team members. Such errors are preventable when following the predefined protocols.

Hospitals should adopt security procedures such as check-list before the surgery as well as the informed consent form, the pre-anesthetic evaluation, the materials needed, the tests available and the involvement of team members. The time-out or final check also needs to be done by a staff member telling aloud the surgical site, patient name and other items that are defined by each hospital before a surgery or invasive procedure.

Goal 5	Goal Requirements
Reduce the Risk of Health Care–acquired Infections	Infections are preventable events, which result in undesirable and additional suffering for the patient and extra costs for the hospital.
Hospitals shall adopt measures to encourage the reduction of infections such as instructing employees to wash their hands properly and regularly, have features such antiseptic hand hygiene, to monitor antibiotic use and create educational campaigns for conscious use of uniforms and sterile materials.	

Goal 6	Goal Requirements
Reduce the Risk of Patient Harm Resulting from Falls	The aim is to reduce and/or prevent the risk of patient injury resulting from falls and avoid the patients falls or control the risks from falls, especially elderly patients or those using medications that make predictable decline.
Hospitals need to assess and reassess periodically the patients likely to fall by eliminating the risks identified. Patients need to be counseled about the risk and when necessary request help from nurses, hospitals needs to maintain some independent lighting at any time, clearing the circulation of the patient and have a safe means for the patient go up and down the bed.	

For the physician or other health care professional, an error can result in civil and/or criminal lawsuit, to unpleasant consequences with the syndicate or organization to which he is registered, and depending on the service provided by professional or by institution also be accountable to the justice.

For the physician the situation may be even more complex because he/she is ultimately responsible for what happens to the patient. It is noteworthy that the physician has no obligation to cure a patient, but to make the possible with the knowledge practice permitted by the medicine, working with zeal and diligence to achieve the cure. That is why the justice in many countries considers the action of a physician as a means and not just an end itself, which could, for example, result in death despite the best and most competent care performed by the health care team. For example, the result of a surgery can be a death, despite all the competent care provided.

When there is a charge of error, it is up to the physician or other health care practitioner to prove that he/she acted properly doing everything in his power or in the medicine to treat the patient. In these circumstances it is the health care professional and the institution who must prove that they acted properly and did not commit any error, due to the fact that the burden of proof to be in favor of the patient and his family. In addition to the expertise and the testimony of other professionals, the informed consent form and medical records are still the main documents used in the defense of claims of errors, which is why the term must be on the record and this should always be updated and filled in correctly by all staff that provide patient care.

Normally health care professionals are aware of the risks caused by incorrect information in the medical records, and the importance that all patient care is registered as well as the results of laboratory tests and all complimentary information, and reported when appropriated. Among other proofs the records need to be filled properly helping to prove the causal link incriminating or excusing the professional. The problem is that some professionals not always see some patient harm situations as critical or reportable as indicated by the Office of Inspector General. According to the OIG the hospital reporting systems do not capture most patient harm[3], with hospitals reporting an estimated of only 14% of patient harms events that Medicare patients experience. The staff did not perceived as reportable the remained 86% of events.

In a report published by an important Brazilian magazine called Veja entitled "They by them", 1119 doctors from an amount of 5200 responded several questions asked. Some of them brought information that allows us to draw a picture of the practice that involves even the errors and failures that can occur in health institutions. In the questionnaires 62% say they have

---

[3] Office of Inspector General - Report (OEI-06-09-00091) 01-05-2012.

never made mistakes or even have hurt the health of a patient, while 38% said yes. About 51% said they would never admit they committed a mistake with their patients, while 39% said they admit when they make mistakes. But what happens when a physician realizes that his colleague was wrong or committed an error? According to the survey:

%	Reaction from the physician colleague
71	Talk to the colleague who made the mistake
11,5	Shut their mouth
8,5	Notifies the hospital or the Regional Council of Medicine
4	Talk to the patient
5	No answer

On the other hand, in the same survey is easy to see that a large number of doctors, about 95% are happy and fulfilled with their work. From the universe surveyed 57% sought medicine because they think they were born to be a doctor and 26% to help people, who denote professional committed with their patients and with the cure of diseases. They are doctors because they love the life they chose. It is very important for those in need of treatment to find out the genuine interest of the physicians to help them, despite all the difficulties they may face in the everyday life. Thanks doctors!

Some words from a Physician:

"There are situations in which there is no treatment and the patient will inevitably die. In such cases, it is the duty of the physician to talk with their family and decide what is best to ensure a dignified and painless end. [...] I'm an oncologist. During my years of medical practice, I had to experience hundreds of times, situations in which there is no treatment capable of reducing a tumor and the patient will inevitably die. In these cases, I think it is the duty of the physician to talk with the family and decide what is best for the patient to ensure a worthy end, without suffering, how to make less painful the last few weeks or months. Only a person utterly insensitive would deny a patient the right to die when life becomes worse than death."

MD. Ezekiel Emanuel

Chapter 5

THE COMMUNICATION IN THE HOSPITAL CONTEXT

The communication is not just a characteristic that distinguishes us from animals, is a link with other human beings, is the balm that we lack in the lonely and more difficult moments, it is through it that we can be heard and listened to both, those who we know or who are strange for us. Communication is essential in all human relationships, personal and interpersonal, resulting in the understanding between the parties. To communicate is as important as knowing how to communicate.

Every day we face different situations in which good communication or the proper communication can solve problems or increase them. Many times we think we understand or we are understood by the other person with whom we communicate, and in fact the message was insufficient or wrongly absorbed. The problems aroused from bad communication can be catastrophic.

There is a story that reflects well the damage from poor communication. A young executive tries impatiently to operate a shred paper machine on the table. A new employee seeing his director in front of the machine without knowing what to do, run to help him, turning on the machine and putting the paper who is being shredded. The director right after delivering the document thanks profusely the good will of the employee and says: − Thank you, this document is very, very important, and for anything in the world I might lose it! Please, I need only one copy. Well, at this point of the communication it was too late. Although it is only a comic story, illustrates well the mistakes that can prevent a good communication, even with the best intentions in human relations. Although the mechanisms developed to ensure a good communication, there is no guarantee that there are no faults or noise in the communication process at some point of time.

If communication is of vital importance in the corporate world, it must reach an even higher level within the hospital environment, where the clarity and precision in which the message is transmitted, can literally mean the difference between life and death. It is not uncommon to see healthcare professionals talk while is writing a report, filling a prescription or performing some important task increasing the risk of failure or error.

In the health care industry we deal with people, human beings. It is important to know how to interact with people, with persons. There is however another factor that affects this whole relationship, the emotional state of those involved in this process who may affect the understanding when the information sent is not the same received. To communicate with the most different people is not easy, especially in hospitals where words with dubious sense can give rise to erroneous or misleading interpretations and generate the worst possible problems. From the moment the hospital advertises its services (does his marketing) to when the patient returns to his home, there is a complex communication system involved in all processes that culminate in their treatment and complete recovery.

It is of vital importance a perfect communication when the patient is in a hospital, a hostile and alien environment to him. Usually lacking information and eager to details, all information offered will be eagerly accepted, especially when offered by medical personnel. These are times that a good communication (rapport) can alleviate the suffering of the patient and reassure the trust among family members. The warm welcome at the reception and admission unit is essential for the patient and his family to feel good and is the hospital business card, and will send the message how will be the service throughout the stay. Words must be measured, not the warmth and attention.

Communication within the hospital between healthcare professionals reaches its critical moment during urgencies or emergencies, during conflicts or even due to personal resistance to express well and clearly when some distortion can occur. As the body also speaks the non-verbal communication is also evaluated by the recipient, body and facial expressions, tone of voice, sighs, and even the eyes can invalidate or contradict any information transmitted.

Good communication involves empathy, because many times the patient can send messages that only a careful eye can catch. The relationships in many institutions, especially those hospitals worried with the quality of the medical care is giving high priority to the quality of the services provided by the hospital staff, exceeding the willingness to understand and make themselves understood. Avoiding mistakes can prevent lives being lost or the occurrence of damages.

For active and independent people to be hospitalized can be a traumatic experience. The loss of autonomy of the body, the transfer of care to someone never seen before, even a recognized professional, in many cases affects the mood and emotional state of the patient who finds himself bathed and cleaned after their physiological needs for hands that are not theirs. So there are patients who respond unconsciously bad to the service as a form of self-protection. The instinct of self-preservation can hurt the professional, without however being that its real intention.

When the patient is hospitalized he often feels powerless during the care. In these circumstances it is very difficult for him/her to open its soul or express the pain he/she feels. The treatment team must be attentive to the language used by the patient to convey what he/she is feeling or looking for. As they cannot always express themselves adequately it is important to pay attention to the body language to capture their feelings, as well as to police itself for not to convey one information and pass another, for example, through facial expressions.

Most common types of behavior observed in hospitals

Passive	Avoid express its concerns, opinions and feelings. Shut up before the caller, asks little and often does not question any advice given. Normally feel helpless and usually submit himself to the guidelines and rules, often feel powerless before the people and the situation.
Aggressive	Usually complain when believes that was not properly helped. He is not a good listener or empathic, is normally an impatient critic, and it is not uncommon to not respect the employees and other customers. Are sometimes verbally or even physically abusive violating the others rights.
Assertive	Are empathetic and communicative individuals, also a good listener. Make the possible to be understood when communicating and seeks to establish a rapport with the caller. Try to interpret the information with other means when cannot understand the message.

The way a person tries to convey the message can be effective or not, depending on how he behaves during the communication, there must be harmony between voice, gestures and content. About 93% of our message is in the form in which it is transmitted and only 7% will be absorbed in the content. This explain why many motivational speakers are more concerned with the presentation format and less with the content. As you can hear in many organizational environments, a lie told with confidence and tranquility is more persuasive than a truth spoken with doubt and without confidence.

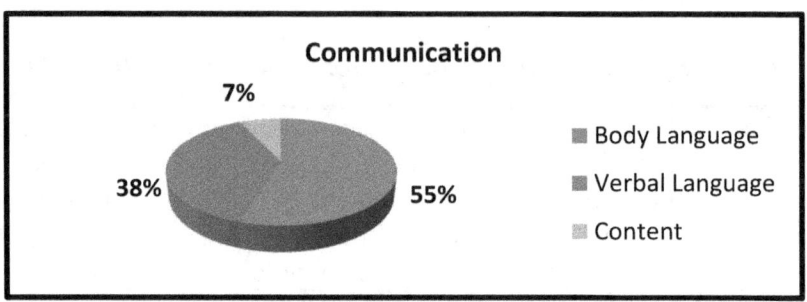

Understanding the communication at hospitals

The job of those who works in health care organizations involves not only the nurses and doctors, but all professionals working within a hospital. Everyone is important and is an actor involved in the process of healing the patient. Having everybody this collective importance in improving patient care, any misunderstanding between an employee and a patient or its family may undermine all efforts improved by other professionals.

The professionals of clerical area, from the front line and those of operational department, besides of the nursing care team, has the important role in assisting the client during the time of physician absence, or about 24 hours of the day, and has based his work in the human relations. The personal contact is the critical moment where the entire institution is evaluated by those who seek it. The voice, body and facial expressions say a lot more or are all the time transmitting messages that even the sender maybe cannot perceive. This means we can say something and transmit other information quite different from what we speak, and can easily be captured by our interlocutors. These are the various forms of communication summarized in verbal and nonverbal ways.

Likewise, the professionals working within the hospital, no matter what its field of expertise or knowledge, must learn to decode the messages sent by the caller no matter if is a patient or a peer. Decrypt messages that someone sends may not be an easy task, especially in difficult times or when overworked. It is essential to try to understand the meaning of the messages the patient send at all times and try to understand their meaning. Also, understand their real needs and establish a bond of mutual trust, to be sure that the message was received and understood clearly.

For someone used to take care of its own body and who feels independent, being hospitalized is a traumatic experience. Do not be understood in their inner needs is terrifying. The loss of autonomy of their own body or the transfer of the care to strangers, may cause profound marks on a person turning their attention to details unseen before. A person who owns their wills do not admit even for a moment to become like a public object, even with the specific care by professionals, without suffering or a change in its behavior or mood.

It's not just the physical problem, only the body that will be affected, but also the emotional side and personal behavior can change during a prolonged hospitalization highly dependent on the staff. It is not pleasant to have someone cleaning up after the physiological needs, or giving daily baths which implies even wash the private parts when the person can't do it by himself.

As it is not possible to separate the psychological side of the physiological, the recovery of some patients may depend much more on the emotional side than just of physical factors. As the emotional side is under stress, the recovery will depend on how he will feel during that treatment, meaning that the feelings of rejection or acceptance will affect their final clinical condition.

To better understand what happens we need empathy and to put ourselves in the same position of the patient. It is an unfamiliar environment where they often do not know exactly what will happen and when. The climate of pain and sadness that permeates many hospitals amplifies the fears and inner fears of death. In this environment the patient will react sometimes unconsciously as a means of self-protection, because it is a strange environment where he may think anything can happen to him. His natural instinct of self-preservation can sometimes hurt the professionals who deal with him without, however to be his real intent.

When the patient is hospitalized, often he feels powerless. In these circumstances, it is very difficult for him to open his heart or to express the inside pain. The healthcare professionals who work directly with the patient must be aware of the language signs used by the patient to convey what he is feeling or wanting. As the patient words can come out hard, they need to pay attention to the body language to capture their feelings, as well as to police itself not to say something and pass other information to the body through gestures and facial expressions.

Making the hospital communication easier

The use of empathy in the professional relationship always tends to favor the bilateral communication. There are ways to facilitate such communication to match the interlocutor and the caller at the time of contact. The person who is talking to a patient or a family should seek to position himself in a similar way to the other person. If the patient is standing, the employee must also stand up to make possible a relationship of equality between them, avoiding the superiority of one over another.

If the person is sitting, the way to cross the arms or touching different parts of the body may be similar with the person in front, but never exactly the same way to do not cause any embarrassment among the patient and staff. This causes in the subconscious of the patient an impression which will lead to a mutual understanding (body language), improving the relationship through the induction process, if done correctly.

Many of the conflicts we experience are due to the image we create from some people, or depending of the situation we create a mental image of the person in front of us. In many instances that unpleasant and demanding person in front of us, is in other circumstances someone sweet and happy. Under stress we all tend to change our behavior and is exactly what happens with many people in hospitals. We have to understand the situation and imagine that the person is having a "bad day" or facing a "difficult time", looking for the situation from another perspective that he is not a "difficult person". Maybe then we will open a window of opportunity to the person realizes where he is exaggerating, even if he does not retract.

In critical moments it is important to show to the person you are trying to understand the situation, to let him speak what he wants and in some cases even encouraging him to expose what he has to say before any answer. This serves as an outlet to vent their feelings and make it more prone to accept another point of view, from the professional or the hospital rules. It does not mean that you are giving reason to the patient who is causing minor or major offenses. To agree with some points in common helps to minimize friction and reduce the differences between the parties. The patient in most cases is not against the employee or the hospital, it is just thinking in himself. The last resort is to listen; it is sometimes what many people need, ears to listen them.

In the daily interactions, the professional working in hospitals regardless of function or department, and especially in those where the patient contact is constant, will find themselves faced with many difficult situations without way out. In these times common sense should prevail. This does not mean to agree with everything the person says or demands.

Everyone should have a definite point of view about everything, and, of course when it comes to standards, rules or a hospital policy there is no way to avoid them. In these hot times it is unhelpful to say that this is how things work or that it is the rule. There are other ways of saying the same thing, without however, to seem offensive and above everything to win the confidence of the patient or the family member.

The first important point is transpiring that you understand the patient or the situation, let him talk and encourage exposing everything that he has to say before replying. This works as a way to let him vent, relieve the oppressing reasons and realize their true motivations. Only after listened someone, you should expose the vision of the hospital or professional involved in the matter.

Again, this does not mean the patient is the victim. Agree with some points in common helps to minimize friction and reduce the distance between the interlocutors.

It is important to remember again that the patient in most cases is not against the provider or against the hospital, it is just trying help himself. Ultimately, even if there is nothing to do at the moment, the employee must present some form of temporary relief as to report that will seek to remedy or solve the problem, even if it is not possible at that moment. This is not a lie to the patient, but a measure to gain some time to think about some way out, or to look for another professional to act at the core of the problem.

Yet, another important issue in communication that helps in daily interactions is the use of words and expressions that can completely change the meaning of what is said, minimizing or maximizing the information. This applies, for example, to the word "but." A surgeon can tell his patient: - The surgery was great, but you will get a scar!" The emphasis here was on the scar despite the most important point is the result of the surgery that was great. The message sent here is that the scar has a greater importance than the surgery.

Let's look at another angle the doctor talking to his patient: - "You will get a scar, but the surgery was great!" The emphasis was on the end of the phrase emphasizing the surgery and not the scar, the patient will always take the maximum advantage of a great surgery that saved his life. The same situation can be observed when saying that a woman is beautiful, but her shoes are dirty. All the beauty fades before the dirty shoes. While saying that the shoes are dirty, but she is beautiful exalt its beauty and becomes the dirty shoes insignificant.

The same goes with our communication with patients, families and other employees. A single word can distort or change the meaning of what we're trying to say. For a patient who has time lying down in a hospital bed to analyze every word of information given to him, it becomes a problem to say thoughtless phrases or pass information who is not authoritative. An only "but" can give reason to numerous interpretations reflecting in the mood of the patient and his family. Other words with the same effect are "if" and "when" that means a sense of possibility and time, something unreal to who counts the minutes to be cured or to leave the hospital.

However, the best way to make a clear and intelligible communication has not changed despite the passing years. As to ask if the person, patient or family understood and ask them to explain back what they understood. In most cases we can see clearly the mistakes that the communication can cause, for better or worse. To ask the peer to repeat what was said is still considered the best way to avoid misunderstandings and avoid unsatisfactory results. After all, if there is noise in the communication even between husbands and wives, with friends, parents or people who enjoy a close relationship and close contact among them, we shall not wait less from people who we simply have business contacts.

The professional who chooses to work in health care industry should be aware that he will acts in a critical area, working with people in situations of fear, stress and sometimes risk. It is necessary to understand the reasons that lead a person to act stupidly. Normally a person is frightened, sometimes with pain and fear of dying. The professional does not need to agree with the person or with his way of acting, but need empathy to avoid entering in his game.

It is more common than we think, but most of us act the same way when we are under pressure, fear or risk of death and we do not always realize it. A simple exercise is to ask our family how we become when we are ill, many will reply that we are grumpy, respond with stupidity or we may have become ungrateful. That is, patients are not very different regardless of whether a doctor, engineer or a businessman. So, the healthcare professional must never expect to see someone coming through the door of an emergency room a lively and bouncy patient saying "Wow! I had a heart attack!" or "Uhuuu! I have cancer!"

Increasingly, patients are aware of their health problems and their rights looking for information before seeking a doctor or a hospital. This search for information has resulted in concerns by many doctors due to the not always reliable source, found on channels like the internet. Part of the problem is in the doctor-patient communication full of technical terms and medicine jargons, hasty and evasive explanations, more yet, in many situations is clearly perceived in the doctors face the dislike and discomfort caused by many questions and inquiries made by patients and their families.

It is not uncommon doctors get angry when a patient comes to the clinic with many questions after searching the internet the information available about his disease. On the other hand, one would not expect anything different if the patient leaves the room or a hospital with more doubts than he entered. It is known that many medical schools encourage the use of technical language even in contact with patients. It creates a communication barrier that hinders the understanding of the actual patient's disease, which often results in other problems, such as difficulty of the patient to follow the medical advice.

Normally human beings cannot retain so much information in situations of stress and fear, which is why doctors need to stimulate the presence of another person who can help if the patient cannot remember the treatment guidance's. With the recognition of the need to move closer to the patient's and speaking its language, the doctor gives a large step toward making the doctor-patient relationship more effective and lasting.

Understanding the conflicts

To understand many of the situations in which we operate, it is sometimes necessary to get out of the environment in which we stand and watch ourselves from outside the box. Watching our interlocutor from above or from outside, can help us to understand the dynamics of what occurs inside the problem. Being inside the situation can distort our judgement sense and decision-making at crucial moments. Dealing with humans at hospitals will make us to act differently in the various moments, sometimes emotionally, sometimes rationally even at the same circumstances.

One way to better understand how this happens can be tried in the activity one where four lines can be used to go over all the points without lifting the pen from the paper. Put the pen over the first point and go ahead drawing the four lines. Do not take the pen from the points, they must be one after another until the four lines were drawn. To reach the solution we have to come out of the situation and from the outside, our enlarged view can find where the answers to many of our conflicts are.

Activity 1

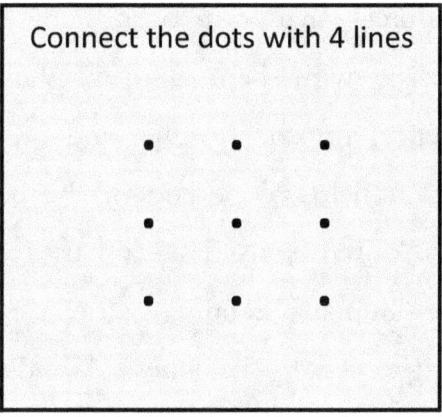

Connect the dots with 4 lines

Note that if we want to connect the dots with four lines is necessary we leave the environment in which the points are, to look from above and cover them with the four straight lines. The activity two follows the same pattern, but now only three lines should be used to unite the six points.

Activity 2

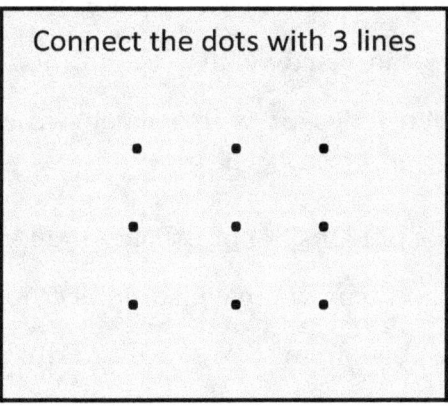

Connect the dots with 3 lines

These exercises give us a dimension of how we should understand the conflicts that can occur not only between employees, but especially with clients and their families, who are the reason of existence, for the hospital and the professionals who work within it. It helps to get rid of the habit of always seeing our rights and our reasons first, and try to understand a little more about the "human" standing before us, with his fears and needs, often frightened by its illness. We do not need to agree, to like the person or to accept what he has to say, but we must imagine how was to be in the same situation or at that moment; to realize the reasons and motivations that led the person to act in any way harshly or stupidly.

Again, it is more common than we realize, but most of us act in the same way when under pressure and we do not even realize. In other words is very common to demand from others a behavior that we not always present in our turn. In short, if we ask our loved ones how we become when we are sick or hospitalized, we can discover that we are not always as polite as we imagine, been equal or worse when we are all in the same situation.

Looking not only inside, but seeing it all with a holistic look, we can understand why we make some decisions at certain times. And based on this premise we noticed that a patient and/or family members are more likely to act unconventionally during tense situations such as hospitalization or death of a loved one. It is very important to establish the goal of being part of the healing process of the patient, to be a healing facilitator or to support those who make possible the healing. It will increase the sense of appreciation and personal achievement, since this becomes the rule and not the exception within a hospital.

Exercises solutions

Activity 1

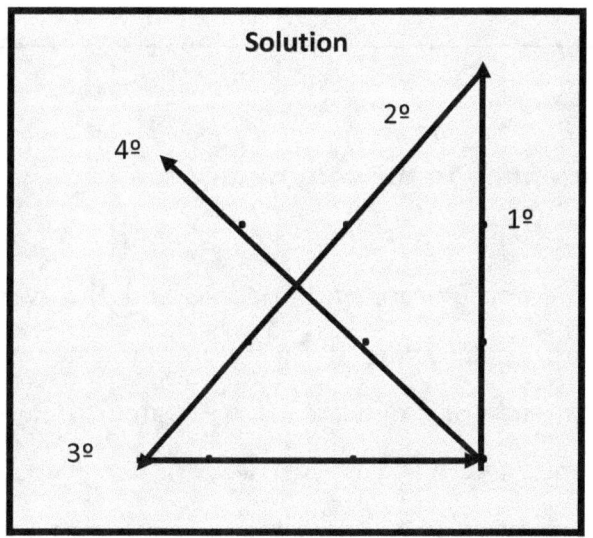

You can see the points here to understand how the exercise works. Follow the numbers and the arrows to from 1 to 4 to accomplish the task. In activity 2, go from above to below, from 1 to 3.

Activity 2

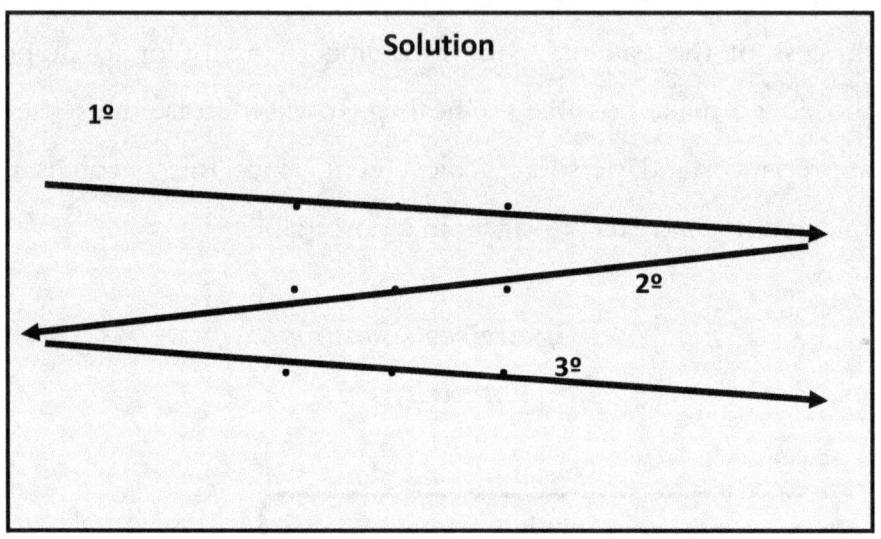

Paying attention to the communication

Every day we communicate with people and the world around us, often without knowing it. We communicate even when we do not want to communicate. If we want to stay in silence, we pass a message to everyone we do not want to communicate or communication is not desired. If we are happy, we send a message that something good happened or is going to happen. If we are sad, the message will be sent the same way. Both the lack of communication and the excess of it can be harmful in the workplace, requiring the professional to police it all the time.

A French newspaper, Impact Médecin (*apud* Meyer, 2002) joked with a situation that has become common in hospitals in different countries. A woman hospitalized for several days complaining about the absence of her physician with a nurse:

"- When the doctor comes to see me? I never saw him.
- But she comes every morning since you arrived.
- Oh! It's a woman? I thought it was a nurse, she never said a word and contented himself only looking at my chart."

While somewhat unlikely to occur, it is important to remember that as much as a word, the silence also speaks a lot about the person. Or can no longer say. All the staff should be aware of the importance of saying at least "good morning", "how do you feel today", "I would be glad if I can help with anything". Others words that can produce good results are compliments, they are not expensive, they will not reduce who offers and make the others day much better.

Among the worst situations that can exist in the hospital, the death is perhaps the most difficult, creating awkward situations for everybody. Most employees do not know yet how to deal with this, and little attention is given to this problem, less yet training. Some employees with his good will try to politely say phrases that often create more problems because of the faith of each one, rather than necessarily help. These are difficult moments that need skilled people to deal with sensitive behavior of rage, anger, grief, violence and even in some cases, relief and joy. Yes, it can happens!

Among the professionals who need training to deal with this situation, are many doctors, due to the nature of their job they still need to know how to transmit the information of "death" to the family. While it may be common for many professionals, the loss of a loved one can be devastating for some people, and how the news is given at this time weighs heavily. Who works with human beings, needs above all, to be human.

Meyer (2002) notes that "the British are organizing medical communication courses (Medical Interview Teaching Association, Cancer Research Campaign and Counseling Communication Research Center)", like many Americans who work the communication of these events to the families"(American Academy on the Doctor and the Patient)." He also notes that:

> *Physicians are not prepared for it. An announcement of death of a son to his parents in an accident made by a Police officer, does less harm than that given by a physician. Women suffering from breast cancer said that, the manner in which the diagnosis was revealed to them*

weighed heavily in their degree of anxiety and tolerance to treatment.

The importance of understanding this moment can be seen by how different cultures view and understand the death, following different rituals. In some religions, some forms of mourning can scare who's next, creating misunderstandings with the unnecessary intervention of security guards. In many situations, the feeling of loss and despair can take hold of the person making it uncontrollable, requiring much skill to calm him/her down, usually by family members.

The communication between employees must also receive attention. It is not uncommon to see employees laugh or talk happily next to places where relatives mourn the death of a loved one, or are awaiting sad medical news, creating an unpleasant situation for the family. Patients who are hospitalized in ICUs, especially in a coma are often seen as unable to hear or understand what occurs in the environment. While happy talks are made, stories are told beside the bed, and unusual other situations occur, silent listeners may not be able to react or do even more, but they can hear and remember later what is being said.

Lucena Junior (1988) while a patient in an ICU after suffering a serious traffic accident, recounts conversations and situations that he heard during his "unconscious" state while he was being treated at a hospital. The fragments of this exciting story, show moments that the author/patient was in some phases of treatment, without the professionals who cared for him to know or realize that, he was conscious and listening everything that was happening in the environment.

Suddenly, the film projection is interrupted. It stopped like a flash, popping. Everything is very cold and dark. I hear noises around me. Was I awake? I try to move and realize I can't. No muscle responds. I still can't move. I try to open my eyes. It seems that are already open. At least I do not feel the movement of the eyelids. But, if it is already open, why I do not see anything? Why everything seems pitch black? The noises are still around. One of these noises seemed to be of a little machine whose motor ran slowly. Another, of bubbling liquid. I set my hearing to those strange sounds. Something tells me I'm awake.

A door is opened and there is a higher noise from people. I hear strange voices and an annoying sound of wheels. It seemed to be of a small table car. I would not know the reason for this noise annoy me so much. It was as if I had heard that noise before. I feel that the table car is placed next to me. People talk. I hear voices of a woman and two men. Discuss something that I could not understand. One of the men thought would be better to wait another twenty-four hours. The other said it was risky. It was better to puncture now. What was a puncture? I do not even know if they were speaking about me. It could be about someone else ... [...]

In a desperate effort, I tried to talk to those people. I could not move my lips. The voice did not exist. It seemed to have a stone in my throat. Something prevent me even to swallow. But I had to talk to them. A new attempt, no success. I could not do any kind of movement to attract attention.

In fact, I neither had time to try again. As if I had received a kind of shock, I felt a piercing pain, unbearable, in the right side of my head. Something like a needle to pierce my brain. It was like a split second. I felt uncontrollable urge to scream, kick and could not do anything. They kept sticking. The despair did not last long. Blacked out.

I do not know how long I stayed off. When I woke up again, I realized I was at the same situation. I could only hear and smell. There were people around me, speaking as talkative. No voice was familiar. The voices weren't the same as before. I hear the door open and, again, the sound of wheels. I shudder with dread. I would face the puncture again? I set my ears and I realize that this noise was different. It was wheels, but it was not like the one before. I felt relieved. I was sweating cold or at least I thought I was. (Lucena Junior 1998, pages 26-28)

As reported by the author and former patient, although it was not noticeable, everything that occurred in the environment was heard and felt. How well or poorly placed phrases may encourage or discourage people who are apparently unaware? How many people are awake and can't move or tell anything for those who take care of them? Can someone imagine how painful is trying to communicate and say "hey, I am alive! Please help-me!" with no success? Only who returned could tell and write about this situation, as this patient did.

Elsewhere the author/patient recounts the moment when a nurse tells that he had "awaken" from the apparent immobility, hearing what was talked and realizing that he was going to face a new surgery.

A huge well-lit spotlight on me, the buzz of many voices and the sound of metal objects put me on alert. I identified the voice of [a nurse] asking the [doctor] about scalpels, tweezers and other tools he would need. My blood ran cold. I would not be examined. I would be under a surgery.

[The nurse] said to the doctors I had woken up a little earlier in the ward. [...] I heard a voice, that later, would become unmistakable to me: "This guy had all the time in the world to wake up and decide to do this right now? [...] I did not find the joke funny. What all time in the world? How long did I sleep?

I heard comments about anesthesia. A shiver of fear went through me. If I sleep forever or black out at once? And if I never wake up anymore? I had only just regained consciousness and managed to communicate with people. It was not fair. There was no longer any doubt. I would even go under the knife. (Lucena Junior, 1998 pages 39, 40)

A few reports in the literature clearly show what happens to patients who are apparently unconscious, according to his own view, in the moments of hospitalization or prior contact with the professionals. Although the author is grateful for the care he received, from white angels as the healthcare professionals seems to be at critical moments, the chapter ends with a touching remark.

> *I imagine that human beings can also experience dire agonies, no worse than that. Is unspeakable the terror that grips the person in a situation of such impotence. To face a brain surgery, against his will and without at least knowing why. To be blacked out without knowing why. To lose the control and be at the others mercy, up to what they want do with you. (Lucena Junior, 1998 page 41)*

No matter where it occurs and how the communication occurs within the departments of a hospital, when near the patient it should always be uplifting, even when the patient is in coma the words can be used to stimulate recovery and to praise. We maybe never will know if it works with the patients who dies, but if yes, will make the last moments of the person much more comfortable than the frozen air conditioning of any ICU. May our words be a balm and part of the healing process, even if we did not know who is listening to us and how our words will take effect.

Research conducted by the Federal University of Juiz de Fora/MG involving 100 doctors and 500 patients, revealing the reasons why patients and doctors seek a second opinion.

Why do **patients** seek a second medical opinion?

50%	Lack of trust in the first doctor
42%	Confirmation of diagnosis (mainly in the cases with risk of death)
30%	Persistence of symptoms

Why do **doctors** seek a second opinion from a specialist colleague?

65%	Doubt in relation to treatment
56%	Doubt about the diagnosis

Chapter 6
QUALITY IN THE HOSPITAL
CONTEXT

The meaning of "quality" is usually subjective and is often perceived differently by people, it is not always easy to measure depending on the activity or industry. A simple example is to deliver a service with 99.9% of quality guarantee. An extraordinary number for a service, when you consider the complexity of the world in which we live. However, depending on area of expertise as healthcare, 0.1% can mean 20 000 wrong prescriptions in a year. A scare number for a quality service.

When we buy a product that we can see, it's possible at some extent to manipulate and measure the degree of strength, durability, color, weight, among other attributes associated with quality. When in use is easier to make sure if the product meets or exceeds the consumer expectations. When it comes to service the situation is quite different, especially those related to health, which are considered intangible and inherently carries the perception of greater risk; due to the intangibility of the results depending on the complexity of the treatment and the patient's perception expected.

For example, in a plastic surgery the perceived quality can vary greatly between the patient and physician point of view. The expectation of the patient may differ from the physician about the outcome of the surgery, leading to conflicts and even dissatisfaction. For a physician can be a good job, but for the patient cannot be exactly what expected.

Unlike other areas, the quality is an intrinsic feature of health activity. The client does not want to be partially cured or accept half of the pain. The goal is to eliminate the disease or alleviate the health problem that cannot be cured, as the pain suffered by a terminally ill patient with cancer. The patient expects that every intervention is to solve the problem and heal the sick, not leaving room for a reasonable service. It makes extremely complex the job of healthcare professionals who works often with unpredictable situations such as bad reactions to a given treatment, emergencies during a surgery, and even the risk of death or permanent damage as may occurs with brain surgery.

With a tangible product we can feel, touch, smell, use again and again, see if it works properly and if meets the needs of the buyer. There is a higher degree of confidence, it is known that if it doesn't work or fail is just to return or request another. With services that is not possible, because the consumption is simultaneous with the production. So, while it is possible to do new tests and make a new surgery, the results cannot be perceived similarly. And the same action cannot be repeated, a new test or surgery will be "another" test or "other" surgery, never experiencing "the same service" twice.

Everybody knows that when is higher the variation in the quality is greater the perceived risk of a product or service. In healthcare is no different, when the opinions among physicians are quite different about the same treatment, the perceived risk for the patient is bigger. The same goes for certain procedures performed in a few hospitals of the world or when there are only a few professionals who perform a certain surgery, it is known that the risks are higher.

The table below shows the perception of risk in products (tangible) and services (intangibles). Bigger the perception of one, smaller the other.

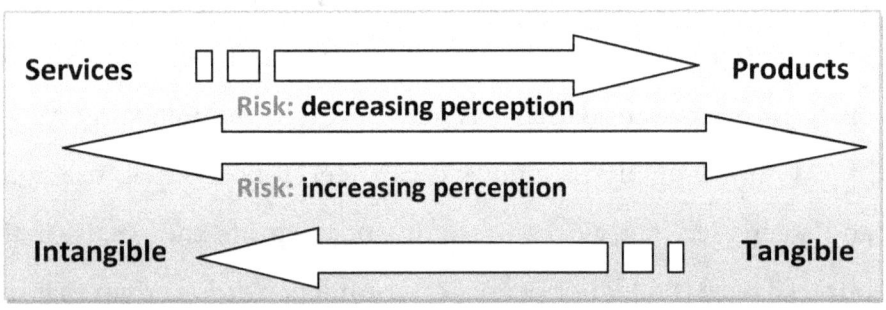

If the perception is difficult to measure and varies from person to person, processes can be standardized to ensure that the optimum result can be achieved. Large hospitals usually have departments which shall ensure that the quality of services and procedures is maintained within the institution, based on indicators and patterns previously established. Among the tools largely used to measure the quality is the PDCA and the Cycle, Plan, Do, Check, Action.

Other useful tools in the quality control are the Cause and Effect Diagram, Pareto Chart and Brainstorming that can be used in a joint or with one complementing the other. The following table shows some tools widely used and its objectives.

Quality tools	Aims
Brainstorming	Create, evaluate and select possible options in meetings or groups.
Cause and Effect Diagram	Search and organize the root causes of problem or situation.
Checklist	Data collection of the possible causes.
Stratification	Grouping of data from a common origin.
Pareto Chart	Line/Bar Graphics showing cause and effects.
5W2H	Questions to find the problems roots cause.

One of the features that can stimulate the quality of service is to promote the contact between the customer with the expected completion of the service in a timely manner, which can be obtained by using indicators. Among the complaints heard in many health services there is a slow response on the time required to deliver the results of the procedures performed. Having a clear agenda is still the best choice always telling the client how long it takes, for example, when the result of a test performed will be available, or how long will it take to clean a room, and so on.

Establishing an effective information system does not create unnecessary expectations and demands. One must keep in mind that waiting is unpleasant, especially when there is anxiety

Non-conformity is not attending, deviation, the refusal or failure to fulfill a specified requirement, accepted standards, rules, practices or conventions.

about the result of a test that will determine the action to be taken. For the healthcare professional is just one more test, but for the patient is a verdict that will affect his life and maybe the future of their family. The vagueness of the answer or ignorance about the patients need are also problematic, especially in an institution that follow certain procedures as an established routine. If someone doesn't know something, the professional has at least to appoint who knows.

Since time is relative between people, half an hour of waiting can be an endless wait depending on the client stress or how it has their needs satisfied. For others, half an hour may be extremely fast. We have to remember that the time of work is different from time of waiting, and that wait is more tiring mentally than when involved in other activities. So, to guarantee an effective assistance, is essential:

➢ Define the services from the patient's perspective

➤ Organize the care based on the solution of the patient's needs

➤ Develop multidisciplinary teams working in unison

➤ To measure the results to accelerate the learning process and apply them in the day-to-day activities

Performance indicators or others data are helpful to assess the quality of services, even for something as subjective as the satisfaction of care, which can be sometimes quantitative or qualitative. It is noteworthy that situations such as excessive complaints or no complaints are, for example, subjective indicators that something is wrong in the institution, the use of indicators will help to detect problems.

To be effective is necessary to know what to measure and how the most appropriate measurement tool will be used, also the use of standardized data to compare. To make the indicators useful it must be produced and used regularly allowing viewing trends over time in the data found. It should also enable local, regional, national and possibly international comparisons, with the results been kept confined or made available to the general public.

Currently the consciousness of rights and what is expected from a product or service has increased among consumers of all social classes in all countries. People are more aware of what they want and what they are receiving. The health care industry cannot afford to produce results with poor quality; quality is an attribute that must be intrinsically linked to life. There should be no margin for error in the case of human lives.

The patient is the main actor of the treatment with problems, desires and expectations differently from each other. Despite the intervention often be as intangible as the result of some surgeries, it is not difficult to measure the degree of satisfaction that is linked to the quality of services delivered to the patient. In other industries the situation is quite different when evaluating a product, a person can know the degree of final quality that is tangible, visible and produces measurable results.

Although the cure of the patient is attributed solely to the physician, and he is the person who holds the knowledge that leads to healing, everyone in a hospital, somehow, participate in the healing process of the patient. So, the quality shall permeate all actions taken within and outside the institution, from suppliers to employees. Every professional plays its role with some degree of motivation while others can be driven by money, others for love, or because the person did not found anything better to work. These opposing energies can directly affects the patient or the way the work is done within the hospital.

The image below shows how the work done by professionals may be sometimes in conflict with the internal and external contingencies, which can range from the efficient care to the lack of structure to work, minimizing or maximizing the benefits the treatment causes to the patient.

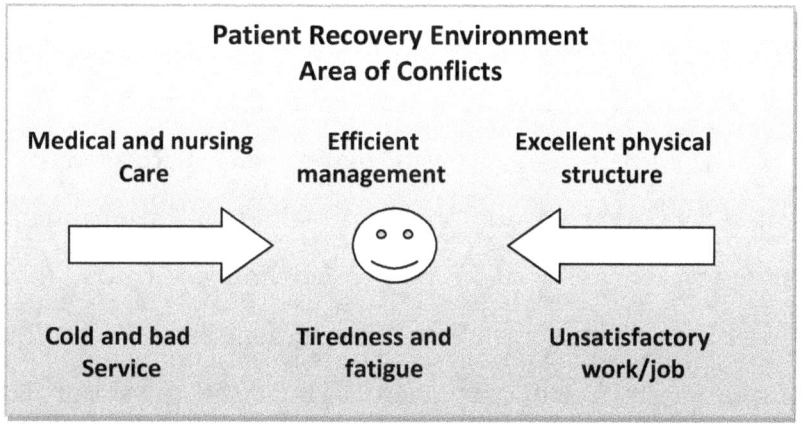

Certification: a commitment to quality in healthcare institutions

The hospital Accreditation or Certification process, whether national or international system, is of utmost importance to ensure that quality of care prioritizing the patient safety through policies, protocols and routines to ensure the best care possible. In several countries the process of quality certification is seen as something common permeating many sectors such as education and health. There is also clear recommendations from government bodies to seek only accredited institutions when going abroad. In other countries the initiative begin with the managers decision to improve patient safety and efficiency of internal processes and routines. It's good for the institution and even better for the patients.

To define and measure quality is extremely difficult, given the intangible nature that it takes for each client, especially in healthcare. The first studies on the quality dates from the 70s and 80s, when Donabedian showed that quality perceived by the patients depended from 30% to 40% of diagnostic and therapeutic capacity, and the higher percentage of 40% to 50% from the relationship between patients and healthcare professionals, especially physicians. Thus, the physician-patient relationship has a high weight in the patient's perception of quality.

There are several international organizations to guarantee the quality in hospitals worldwide, besides each country has its own bodies or national organizations that certificate the quality inside hospitals. Accreditation is a process used by healthcare organizations to implement quality management in the services it provides to their public. It is a voluntary process to which institutions are submitted and are evaluated by an external organization. The hospital accreditation has been seen as a means of ensuring that hospitals meet a set of measures established and defined as best practice by accrediting bodies. When a hospital have an accreditation seal, means to the patient he is in a place where he can trust, that follows internationally recognized protocols and the best practices in medicine. It means safety.

Some of the major accrediting and certifying organizations in the world:

	Certifying Organization
JCI	Joint Commission on Accreditation of Healthcare Organizations
EFQM	European Foundation for Quality Management
QHA	Trent Accreditation (United Kingdom)
ISQua	International Society for Quality in Health Care
IQG	Health Service Accreditation (Instituto Qualisa de Gestão)
ACHSI	Australian Council on Healthcare Standards International
HIQA	Health Information and Quality Authority
UKAS	United Kingdom Accreditation Services
COHSASA	Council for Health Service Accreditation of Southern Africa
CHKS	Comparative Health Knowledge Systems
ONA	Organização Nacional de Acreditação
TJCHA	Taiwan Joint Commission on Hospital Accreditation
HAS	Haute Autorité de Santé
NCQA	National Committee for Quality Assurance
ISO	International Organization for Standardization
ITAES	Instituto Técnico para Certificação de Instituições de Saúde
CCHSA	Canadian Council on Health Services Accreditation
CBA	Consórcio Brasileiro de Acreditação

Each organization chooses the system that best suits its size and budget, due to the costs involved. As a result, institutions that pass through this system of quality assessment, belongs to a select group of hospitals with its quality standard recognized nationally and internationally, including being recommended by governments, health insurance companies and other health institutions from other countries or regions. It is a key differentiator for hospitals that wish to be recognized in the market for their services, and still attract a qualified international demand.

Healthcare organizations certified receive a "certificate" with limited duration, usually two to four years and may be renewed after the expired period. In most countries, the international system with great acceptance and adopted largely is the Joint Commission International. There are other ways to assure the quality used in hospitals not always related to the accreditation process, used largely by departments as the ISO norms (International Organization for Standardization). Sometimes the institution prefers to certify just a process, a product or a department, and ISO fits well in the needs.

There are usually risk assessment that have no direct relationship with the patient, known as "non-clinical" as the physical structure, the waste management policy, air-conditioning system and other equipment, medical gases and other risks such as risk of fire. The "clinical risk" involves the direct or indirect action made by professionals who deals with patients, that is characterized by absence or deficiency of policies or actions in providing the right service to the patient.

Regardless of the system adopted by the healthcare organization, it is a voluntary act. So, it is recognized in the healthcare industry that, the pursuit of quality by a health care institution is a clear and unequivocal commitment to quality. Something that should permeate the whole segment and raise the awareness of healthcare professionals. After all, they deal with the most precious asset of a society, the human life.

Among the quality assessment services, there are those used at hospitals by professional clients, without the employees to know who are evaluating them, just becoming aware that they are constantly being evaluated. Using the services of a mysterious client (mystery client) or members of the board who are less well known, prevents some form of differentiated treatment and fairness in the assessment from the employees. External evaluators in the position of the patient can assess the services by creating situations that range from simple to complex, according to the ability of each employee. Similar situations may occur, however, with customers in other areas. Unscheduled internal audits also help to point out improvements to be adopted and the increase professional awareness of their responsibilities.

There are other

> The first hospital outside the USA to receive an accreditation on medical and hospital care by the Joint Commission International (JCI) was the Albert Einstein Hospital, situated in Brazil in the year of 1999.

methods of evaluation conducted by telephone and questionnaires, quantifying how many patients would return to the hospital if they needed further medical care, or what reasons would discourage the return. A good after marketing survey can correct some distortions and work the improvements before any damage may occur. One of the best way of gathering information is just inside the hospital, in the base of the pyramid. Though neglected, the front-line employees know the main problems and often know the best solution for them, having no conditions to implement or even do not wanting changes that may affect its routine.

It is very common senior executives make plans and create management strategies to be used by the managers, neglecting some main actors that are part of the process. To invite former patients, front line employees involved in the care or assistance and suppliers to provide feedback on services, can show improvement opportunities or their excellence. Listening to those who purchase the service, can generate an amount of new information that will be useful in the analysis of the routine care,

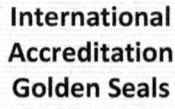

International Accreditation Golden Seals

Joint Commission International – JCI

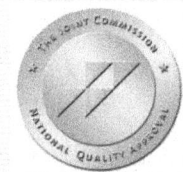

Canadian Council on Health Services Accreditation - CCHSA

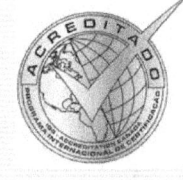

with situations or problems that may go unnoticed resulting in the reduction of quality.

Improving the quality of services often require more employee commitment and attention to the work, affecting some from their comfort zones. However, these are problems easy to be solved, when brought to attention the improvements in the environment reducing absenteeism or high staff turnover, very common at hospitals. Also, changes the attitude of healthcare professionals to not deal with clients in an automated manner, to be aware and supportive rather than hard and indifferent. Dealing with people is not easy, but can be rewarding if it is pleasurable for both sides, for the professional and the patient.

Measuring the quality of services offered to the patients will make the hospital more concerned to what was delivered. Among the major reasons for complaints are poor service followed by unsatisfactory medical treatment. A study conducted in United States resulted in the following data about the reasons why patients do not return to the same hospital.

Percentage and reason for the patient non-return to the hospital	
68%	of patients felt poorly treated at the hospital
14%	of patients were dissatisfied with the services
9%	of patients have migrated to the competition (other hospital)
5%	of the patients sought alternative treatments
3%	of patients have moved
1%	of patients died

Source: Mezomo (1995)

Health care is an economic industry that does not seem to face lack of customers, even with economic crises that reduce the demand in other areas. Currently, the people growing health concern, the return of old diseases, new diseases, emergencies or the improvement in existing treatments seems to raise the number of patients looking for help at hospitals. However, few managers estimate the costs resulting from the loss of customers or the cost of lost services. The loss may be mild and result from an email answered, an unanswered or not returned call, or when the service provided was rudely or indifferently. Many customers who are not linked to the hospital will migrate to other place.

The non-governmental organization SCORE® specializing in market orientation, conducted a study about the damages employees can cause to the company, just for not deliver an adequate service.

• It costs five times more to attract a new customer than to keep an existing one.

• An employee of lower rank may make the company lose more customers than any other senior official could attract.

• 91% of dissatisfied customers will never again purchase any product or service with the same company.

• Dissatisfied customers will tell on average from 8 to 16 people about the purchased product or service received, while 10% of dissatisfied customers will talk to 20 people.

• On average, for every customer who complains about 26 others will be silent.

• If the company acts repairing the bad service provided, on average of 82-95% of dissatisfied customers will do business with the same company once again (Service Recovery).

To calculate the amount invested, the amount of new customers attracted and the cost of lost customers will help the manager to have a safe and reliable indicator in everyday decision-making. Initially, the manager needs to identify what motivated the client to look for the hospital or to leave the hospital. Some marketing campaigns use ads in magazines, television and newspapers to attract new customers. Others are referenced by insurance providers and there are patients who use the hospital indicated by the medical practitioner.

Marketing campaigns that attracts a few customers can be as costly to a health institution, as to see many of its own customers looking for another institution because they did not like the service provided. Some health care institutions pay more attention to bring new clients than to keep the existing ones. A big mistake, both strategies are very important.

Customer loyalty has been a major challenge for any company, even to health care facilities. The hospitals take advantage of patient dependency of a treatment in a given hospital, from one specified doctor or the technology as Gamma Knife existing in a few places. With the plethora of new clinics and hospitals in the market, a client can opt for other professional or a better hospital, to change the treatment or use alternatives as travelling to another country. The competition changed the environment of hospitals and added value to services, with hospitals offering a superior structure than those traditional.

By investing in the quality of its services, the hospital is investing in improved customer service, keeping the old and attracting new clients, innovating and trying to become a model for other hospitals, the hospital will stand longer in the market. The perception of quality in the healthcare industry, not only will retain the client when he thinks to return, as will be pointed to a standard of efficiency when it is quoted by the market.

The mystery client in healthcare services

James Hunter in the book "The Servant" through a simple story, yet powerful, shows that the majority of employees know they in fact work for his boss and company CEOs, and not necessarily for the customers. Despite so many books has been written and taught in courses, that the customers should receive the priority and best attention, mostly staff of large corporations know by practice that their bosses is who can fire them, and usually not the clients. Dr. Lawrence Peter in his book "The Peter Pyramid" addresses this reversal on client attention very common in modern business, even in hospitals, with staff being in the service of a minority within a company and not for the patients.

Therefore, the first major change must come from managers, from team leaders, from the top executives at the hospital. As the learning process is constant, no leadership can afford the luxury of not attending classes and periodic training within or outside the hospital. It's not about where the world has become dynamic, but all areas of knowledge are following the same pace. Moreover, with the many distance learning courses ranging from short courses to postgraduate degrees, no one can argue that he cannot study or update.

Many professionals can have the perception they are doing their best or are delivering the care with quality. However, a conflict may exist in what is the ideal assistance or service, based on the perception of each person or each provider, varying widely. Especially with those hospitals or departments with charismatic or warm people, where is easy to confuse quality with friendly relationship. Some questions need to be made, such as "Are we actually offering the service that our customers really want? Our customers are enjoying the services we are providing, and shall return or tell to others? Are we providing services in accordance with best market practices?"

It is important to evaluate the responses, avoiding taking into account only the long time customers of the hospital, and also focusing on that client with no commitment with the institution. Old customers will help based on previous experience with the services, while new customers have a critical opinion since they are unleashed by the institution and use other hospitals.

A tool used very successfully in several business and often in successful companies is the Mystery Shopper or Mystery Client. This is usually a quality audit of the customer service, where a professional use the products or services of one company without their employees to know they are being evaluated. The action can be performed by a member of the company that is unknown, by managers, by phone or by hiring an outside company. The service has the advantage of recognizing the work of the most competent employees, to train unproductive employees and to detect flaws or gaps in client care.

Many hospitals spend small fortunes with printed materials, training, marketing initiatives and media coverage without, however properly assess if the care provided by each professional is exactly what was advertised. For some companies the service is good if statistically the complaints are below the average for similar services or companies. In the healthcare industry to lose a customer could represent a few hundred to tens thousands of dollars. From a simple medical care in an emergency room to a highly complex surgery, a single customer lost may represent a high cost to the hospital, especially if there are options to influence this and others customers to look for another service.

Upon receiving the results, it is up to senior management to define the strategies that the institution should follow for improvement, and avoid to find scapegoats when problems are detected. Showing the flaws in a positive light and with a focus on continuous improvement there is more adherence to increase the level of service. An efficient way of dealing with quality customer service is using the existing programs of care and patient safety or training courses for healthcare professionals. The actions must permeate all levels within a hospital, mainly involving physicians and nursing staff, as a benefit and not as an obligation or a spare work.

Chapter 7

LUXURY AND COMFORT AT
HOSPITALS

Comfort and luxury are relative concepts generating definitions and interpretations that may vary according to the culture, education, time and the society to which a person belongs. One famous and worldwide known architect usually says that luxury is to have free time to stay at home with the family, for others it can be to live in a mansion, to have a private jet or to own a private island. What is not always discussed is the expanding number of people who had access to the luxury market in recent years enabling them to acquire goods and items previously restricted to an even a smaller portion of people worldwide.

The luxury market may face setbacks in some countries, but not necessarily in a global context as seen in recent years despite the recent economic crises that have hit the world since 2008. According to the 2017 Global Wealth Report, The millionaires rate of growth for the next five years is 54% in Brazil and 73% in Africa, while the world average will be 22%. Only those whose assets are eligible for accounting (considered millionaires) will increase from 36.5 million to 44 million new millionaires (estimated wealth in dollars). In Brazil, they will increase from 164 thousand to 296 thousand new millionaires by 2022 (counting a minimum of one million dollars per person). The fact is, there are more millionaires than is possible to map, due to legal and tax issues. Some fortunes are hidden or spread among families to avoid high taxes.

Even in times of crisis, as has occurred in several countries, the number of people with increasing purchasing power is increasing rather than decrease as dictated by common sense. One explanation is that the money does not disappear in times of crisis, it only changes hands. Nowadays, people in some developing or emerging countries have a higher Purchasing Power and free money to spend, than many people in rich countries largely indebted. Another important point is, despite the crisis that is affecting many countries in the world the number of millionaires has increased in virtually all countries, with the transfer of resources between individuals, companies and countries.

With this change in the economic scenario of many countries and more people having access to the consumption of luxury items, also changed the idea about these countries and the lifestyle they have. In countries like China, India, Brazil and Russia there are now more companies with more than a thousand employees or with annual revenues of millions of dollars than before. These are people who have or are willing to charter a jet to travel to Paris or London, or traveling only in first class and staying in hotels like Claridge's or The Berkerley in London, or at the Ritz or Le Maurice in Paris.

Still, despite the international crisis, the number of people with high incomes (High net worth individuals - HNWIs) or more than one million dollars has increased from 2010 to 2018, as shown in the figures quoted by the British magazine The Economist in 2018. (Number of people with at least $ 1m in assets)

Country	Number of HNWIs per 1000 people in 2018
USA	10.1
Japan	13.6
Germany	11.3
China	0.4
Britain	7.3
France	6.3
Canada	8.4
Switzerland	31.4
Australia	8.8
Italy	2.8
Brazil	0.8
India	0.1

Some of these people have on the walls of their house or apartment paintings by Di Cavalcanti, Portinari, Salvador Dali, they drive Ferraris, wears a $ 50,000 watch and a $ 7,000 dress. Common to all human being who get sick, they do check-ups and are admitted to medical treatment, or to face a surgery in a hospital. At this point, there is a noticeable difference from the hospital environment and poor hospital accommodations, to the comfort they are accustomed at their homes. This difference creates a gap that has not been filled by the Spartan hospital structure focused only on treatment and disease. Despite the mindshift in recent years with the introduction of better hospital structure and hospitality services, most hospitals are still slow to adopt better strategies to attract and treat these kind of patients.

It is not about driving attention to the customers who pay in cash or have a full coverage health insurance and disregard the less fortunate. Medical treatment is the same regardless of the structure or luxury and comfort offered by a hospital when life is at risk. Unlike what many people may think the healthcare does not change in most countries if a patient is rich or poor when life is at stake, what changes is the infrastructure to support these patients. Many people do not realize that the doctors and healthcare professionals who work in top hospitals also can work in public hospitals. Although, is expected that some people prefer to pay more to have a differentiated service, and it is natural they receive a "Premium Service" when they pay more for it.

Despite the high luxury market booming in the main capitals of several countries such as Sao Paulo in Brazil and Beijing in China, hospital managers have not yet realized the importance of providing a superior service to meet this kind of customers. While the goal of hospitalization is the medical treatment, the provision of a structure of comfort and luxury adds value and makes the product "cure" sold by the hospital more attractive. It is not because the patient is sick or just their disease must be treated. Including additional services, a better concierge support and comfort will make the stay less painful, less stressful and will ease the period of hospitalization.

Some people has doubt about the hospital with this structure and range of services, to be considered like a hotel. But, it is exactly this structure of hospitality that will make the treatment more comfortable. Culturally, for many people there is a prevailing thought that those who are sick only need bedding, medical treatment and medicine. Any additional request may be considered an annoyance, generating an association of the patient who wants a little more comfort during their convalescence with a person too much demanding.

There is nothing wrong to treat the patient like a king or queen in one of the toughest moment of his life, when is sick. If these service do not make possible to the patient to recover earlier, can at least give to him/her the best recovery time of their life. As the treatment itself will not differ greatly from one hospital to another, is the hospitality service which plays an important role in attraction, retention and patient care.

The table below show some products and services already consumed by Brazilians costumers, with the prices paid in the country. The price is usually higher than other countries, as USA, due to the high government taxes over luxury imports.

Product/Service	Prices*
Gulfstream G550 Private Jet	US$ 60 millions
Phenom 300 Private Jet	US$ 14,3 millions
Bugatti Veyron 16.4 Grand Sport	US$ 4,7 millions
Ferrari 458 Italia	US$ 1 million
Lamborghini Gallardo LP 550-2	US$ 750 000
Boat Azimut 53 - Azimut	US$ 3,2 millions
Gèrald Genta Collection Watch- Chronograph Rose Gold	US$ 105 000
Boat Targa 58 Gran Turismo	US$ 1,1 million
Richard Mille Watch – model RM011	US$ 70 000 (from)
Female Watch, yellow gold, with diamond ring – Rolex	US$ 55 135
Watch Yacht Master II Yellow Gold - Rolex	US$ 53 560
Textured gold fountain pen - Montblanc	US$ 25 143
Hermés Birkin handbag crocodile	US$ 80 000
Louis Vuitton handbag of crocodile skin	US$ 52 500
Dress in silk and lace - Givenchy	US$ 4 880
Linen jacket - Roberto Cavali	US$ 4 840
Leather Sandals - lanvin	US$ 2 714
Royal Suite - Plaza Athenée (Paris) daily	€ 22 000
Imperiale Suite - Hotel Ritz (Paris) daily	€ 13 650
Bernstein Suite - Hotel de Crillon (Paris)	€ 8 200
Suite decorated by Diane Von Furstenberg – Hotel Claridge's (London) daily rate	€ 11 000
Bottle Perrier-Jouët Belle Epoque Blanc de Blancs 2000	US$ 3 600

Prices may vary according with the country, date and taxes.

Thus, the perception a person have about the luxury services, he can have about the hospitality services too. It can differ greatly in various cultures around the world, from the warm welcome received, something intangible; to the infrastructure and the facilities, something tangible. Hospitality involves a wide range of services and actions, requiring a physical structure dedicated to the comfort and well being connected to the act of receiving, to take care and being hospitable.

The hospital bed is only a detail

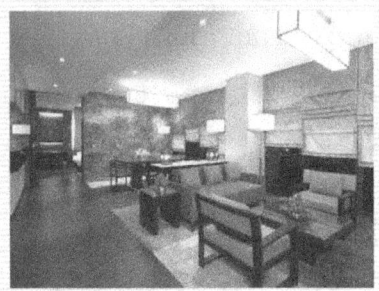

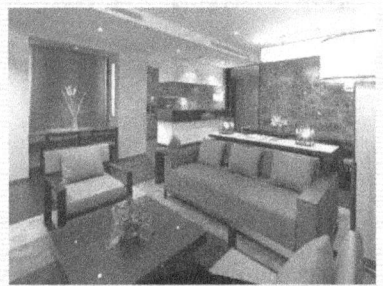

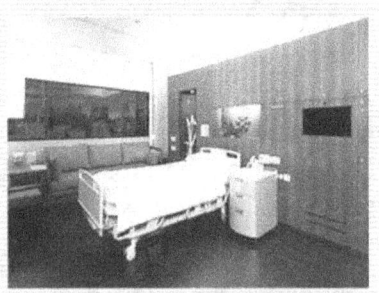

Source: Bumrungrad Hospital

The quantity and quality of services that have been added in the relationship between hospitals and the client over the years, have created a new environment that would enable a person to feel so good or better yet than in its own home. If this set of activities and services has become important in the business world in moments of leisure and relaxation, should not be different within the hospital environment.

In recent years, after many studies done, we realized how much the environment affects positively or negatively the process of recovery of the patient within a hospital. Today is not enough, just to offer a bed and treatment to meet the need for recovery of the human being, as it was a few decades ago where the cure was the only concern at hospitals. The insertion of new professionals in the hospital environment, the discovery of new treatments, the change of mentality with spontaneous search for improvements, corrective body's surgery and the growing

Rooms can be lighter, have big windows, be colorful and well decorated

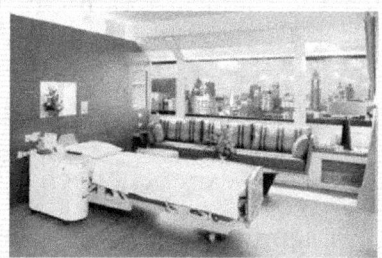

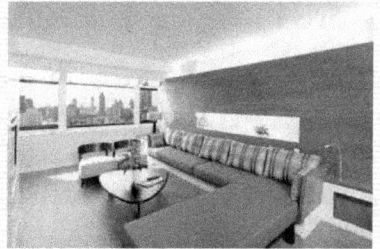

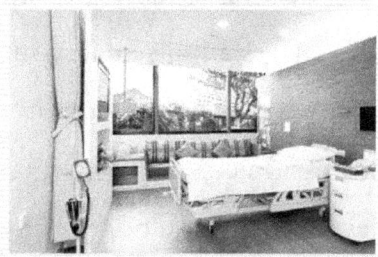

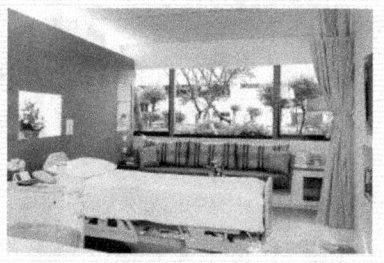

Source: Bumrungrad Hospital

importance of other services have stimulated the patient adherence to treatments, contributing to a better hospital image.

It is expected that the hospital currently can offer more than just the medical treatment. Respecting the differences, the same way a person goes to a store to purchase clothes and enjoys an air conditioning system, bottled water, coffee and other services that make the experience enjoyable; a patient can expect hospital complementary services that will make the stay, that can last days or weeks, more enjoyable. Thus, the care provided by the concierges and care team needs to fit and adjust to the needs of the patient. This means that not all patients are equal, some want to talk and vent, while others prefer a fast and direct service.

Although many hospitals in different countries, mainly in Asia offers a high quality service, with spaces designed exclusively for the patient making it much easier the work of healthcare professionals, there is great resistance in other countries to develop high-standard units with luxury and comfort. It is expected the best service when a person is well and enjoying full health, so it would not be different when someone is sick.

The change begins with the hospital architecture becoming patient-centered thought, and making life easier for the professionals working within the building without being a project full of rooms and administrative sectors, which may be beautiful, illuminated by natural light, to have sculptures, fountains and gardens, yet continue to be a hospital.

There is a considerable change with private hospitals offering additional services to their clients, removing the sad environment that still permeates many public and private hospitals. Part of this change is not linked solely to money, which is the biggest excuse of the authorities to improve the public health system, but the management skills of managers and other professionals committed to build a better hospital. Moreover, it is possible to offer a comfortable structure that is at least clean and based on human respect that does not require any additional money invested.

The importance of the environment and physical space in hospital facilities

What is for many managers just an empty room that would be better occupied by some department, can be for the patient, caregivers and visitors islands of tranquility where they can expect a new information or interact with others, reducing or minimizing the characteristic of hospital-company that some healthcare institutions have. What is considered by some as merely unimportant, can be seen by others as a complement to the patient support structure that helps to increase the peace of mind when entering the institution.

Although the treatment and the cure is essential, items that add value as places beautifully decorated and comfortable contribute to the patient and their families to feel better and cared for. If the hospital make the best from the moment of arrival, the patient tends to believe that the care will continue throughout the treatment and stay. The effect can be seen in the figure below which shows how the structure of hospitality may affect the patient's perception of the place and increase the adherence contributing to the recovery process.

Impact of a good structure of hospitality in hospitals

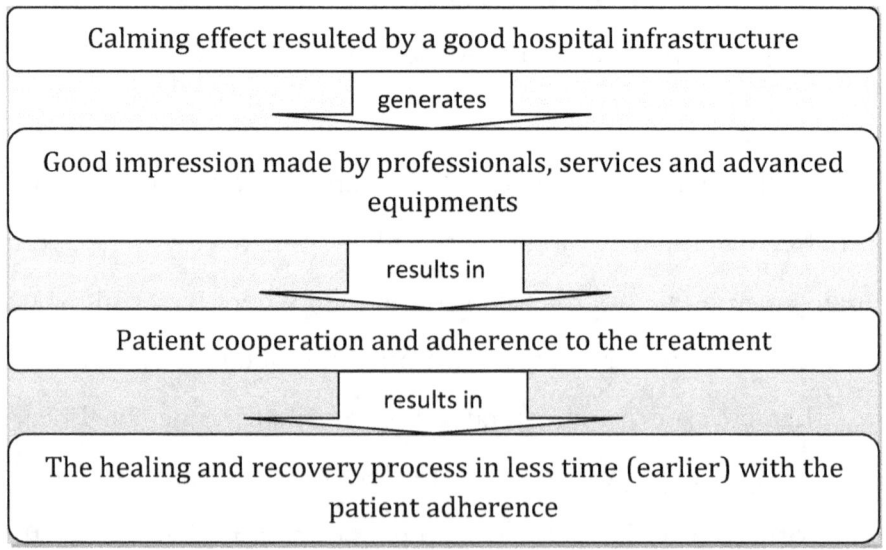

How does it works? Upon arriving at the hospital the client has its car parked by valet, is received by the doorman, while the messengers carry the luggage and handbags, leading them to the waiting room and check-in. The check-in shall be fast, and when dealing with differentiated patients or VIPs, the admission process can be performed on each patient's room. Keeping the privacy and satisfaction.

Authorizations, forms, papers or the documents can be printed anywhere, even on the patient ward. Of great importance, an employee can explain how to use the different services and give others instructions, as well as, the proper handling of equipments. This is also one of the advantages of the messaging service in hospitals. Many hospitals are investing in valuable equipment to customers, without however having

Lively shared room — ward

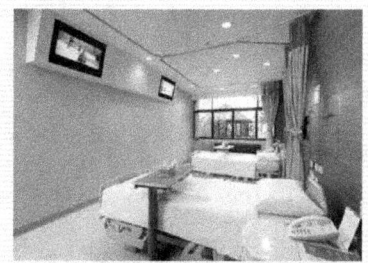

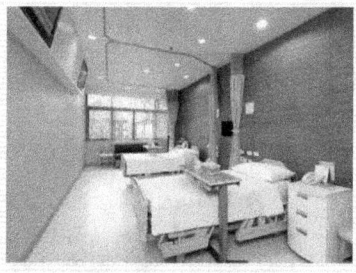

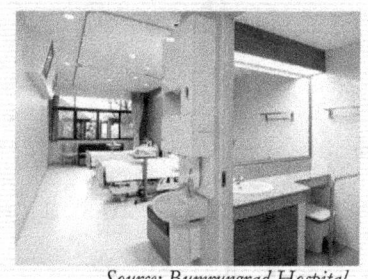

Source: Bumrungrad Hospital

professionals who assist them for guidance and proper use, reducing damages of such equipment.

The hospital room is more than just a recovery place

The treatment must be accompanied by regular visits from the hospitality staff that can ascertain the needs and demands of any patient or their caregivers. After treatment, the check-out follows the reverse routine. Can be performed inside the apartment and the patient discharge without the public attention, resulting in comprehensive care to clients and their families at all times of hospitalization.

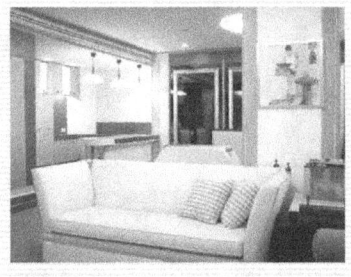

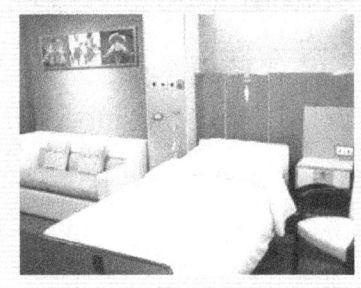

Source: BNH Hospital

The patient may be contacted by the hospitality team after returning home, to check how the service was performed and to use this information to improve future services. In many cases, the check-in or admission process and the check-out or discharge may cause a much deeper impact into the patient's perception than many events during the hospitalization. If failures occur during the service, does not mean that everything is lost, but there will be an opportunity to reaffirm the quality of services provided through an immediate and effective recovery of the client (service recovery).

Providing new services and enabling a smooth transition of all stages is a great merit that the hospitality system brought to the hospitals, as the flow of activities that follows presented in a simplified manner for better understanding of the process.

Simplified view of the flow in the hospitality industry within the hospital

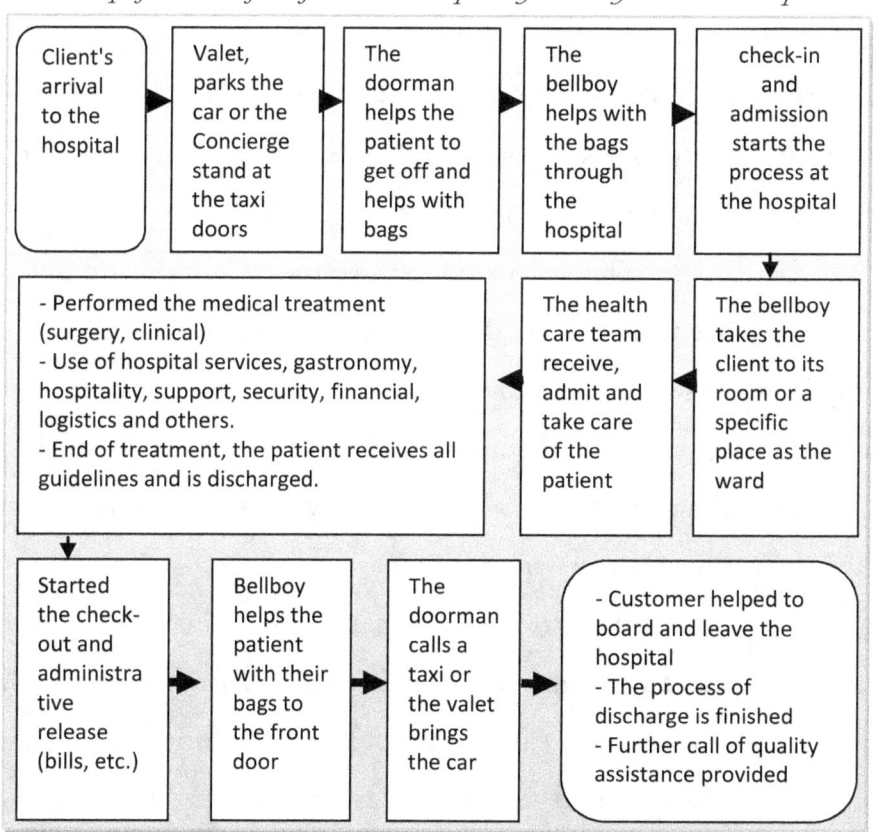

Much more can be done to make the hospital environment more pleasant, as to innovate and decorate each floor with different colors and furniture. The standardization used to keep one color and the same visual style in many hospitals is confusing and does not help patients and their families who can feel lost easily. Wards differentiated by color, clear numbers, images, floors directions and signs not only help patients and visitors, as well as employees reducing the feeling of the same visual environment everywhere. It is possible to move around from one ward/unit or floor noticing differences of the nursing stations and corridors, making much more pleasant the stay for patients and healthcare professionals. A good project can make a huge difference in the perception of clients and staff.

Usually hospital environments are too sober, square units, heavy structure with little gardens and green spaces. There are too many corridors with artificial lighting, rooms without windows and very few lounges and some other spaces are usually small to hold a consultation or treatment, hardly ever used for interaction between family members and visitors.

Hospitals seems to have the same color on walls, with a few or without any bright color, without lively frames or panels and is still very rarely to find some sculpture. Indoor gardens are very well accepted and create an escape from the company pattern that usually permeates the hospital environment, especially if the lighting is natural. The aim of the physical structure of the hospital should be not to isolate the patient and all others in a square box, but welcome and make them feel good and comfortable.

Many lounges are enclosed within four walls with a TV and some pictures to ease the tension of waiting bad or good news. Spaces in front of gardens with natural light generally create a better sense of ease and reduce the anxiety of waiting. Even old buildings can use this strategy creating balconies hanging gardens. Creativity in designing spaces differentiated by type of decoration and colors helps those who spend many hours or days in a hospital.

The walls of many hospital corridors are empty and monochromatic. It could get decoration, artificial lighting if there is no natural and brighter colors making it less stressful to people within the hospital building. The idea that everything must be practical and without differentiation leads to lack of creativity, making some professionals to believe that the soft colors on the walls will have a bad effect over patients who spend minutes or hours in the hospital.

A major concern of the healthcare manager should be on impact and responsiveness that the patient will have when entering the hospital premises. The first visual impression the clients have when arriving will tell them much about the institution. Usually the patients tend to rely more on hospitals with a bold architecture, spacious lobbies and waiting rooms and a structure of imposing size. Transmits to the customer security and tranquility, also transmit the message that if the hospital invests in architecture and infrastructure, also invests in cutting edge technology and most important, has the best professionals. There is a qualitative association of elegant space with a high level of services offered. It is no coincidence that this kind of institutions attracts the most renowned and recognized professionals in the market, and they want to work in these places.

Spacious and airy environments well lit preferably with natural light, with a hospitable staff, high quality service tends to be well positioned in the market and attract a highly qualified demand. The shortage of space that can be transformed into waiting rooms has always been a problem for the vast majority of hospitals worldwide, especially if the goal is the interaction between patients and visitors. For each free space will always be a new business or a new need, meanwhile hospitals become true giant boxes crammed with departments, offices and little space that can turn into square livings.

It is normally unnoticed in most hospitals, but professionals responsible for the decoration insists on keeping entries and access doors confusing to those who does not belong to the hospital environment. The decoration of these spaces with colored panels, different lighting, images etc. make the entrance easy to be memorized, as well as enjoyable. Even the hospital departments such as plastic surgery, an operating room and other accesses can have beautiful doors or entries.

It is not uncommon to observe patients in some hospitals doing his morning walk on the floor where they are hospitalized, while other hospitals use successfully parks and gardens bathed by the sun, even for a few moments or under the watchful eye of the medical staff. It creates a space within the hospital with the necessary security to the patient recovery. This space can be built even on the terrace of the hospitals (sky or roof gardens), normally occupied by machinery, and may receive wooden panels to cover the walls, gardens to cover the raised floor and becomes green terraces.

Although there are discussions about the importance of humanization and the hospitality services, few professionals risked daring to go beyond the orthodox positions assumed by the majority. A unanimous vote is not always a smart option that stifles innovation and creativity to transform the environments and bring more life to the pleasant indoor and outdoor spaces of a hospital.

It is possible to address many topics and describe many different areas of hospitals in several countries that are innovating the hospital environment, serving as a model for managers who are reluctant to accept the new as part of the innovative concepts that are becoming a reality. To let others take the lead awaiting the results and then decide whether it is worth investing, while holds themselves with obsolete and outdated paradigms can result in loss of competitiveness and to lose market share.

In a globalized world, the competition is not necessarily just next to the hospital door and may be elsewhere in the world. If a country wishes to become a destination for international medical high-level service it needs more than simply having qualified professionals, must also invest in the structure of hospitality, services and infrastructure.

While it is indisputable the fact that medical treatment is the main goal for a patient searching for a hospital, the doctor is the most influential person in the hospital environment and who holds the knife, as usually said. The technology is a differentiator that will bring more security to the patient in this decision process. Other factors may affect the patient decision to go or not for a hospital, as the structure of hospitality that can give the necessary support, so that everything else works perfectly and make the patient stay so nice that they will provide good testimonials when discharged.

The hospitality services as a differential
inside the hospital

It is well known in the healthcare industry that economic and social development of a country also leads to changes in the nature of the diseases presented by the population. Problems such as leptospirosis, intestinal worms, malaria, dengue citing common to tropical and developing countries give way to heart disease, cancer, neurological diseases and others in more developed countries. The improvement in economic conditions of a country has an impact on families that alter their standard of living by contributing to the increase of problems related to factors as obesity, alcohol and drugs, also increasing the cost of some treatments and the flow of new people seeking medical care and hospital treatments.

Within the hospital environment, the technology and constant advances in medicine allow doctors to have access to modern resources and equipment, providing patients with diagnoses more accurate and faster healing with less time of hospitalization. Medicine exists between two extremes, the high technology equipment with advanced techniques and the conservatism of medical practice based largely on studies and research. Although this is the reason of the existence of healthcare institutions, the medical treatment has become a commodity that can be purchased almost anywhere on the planet with the same degree of accuracy and quality. A patient may begin his treatment with a doctor in a country and continue it with another doctor in another country without major implications, as it already occurs worldwide with medical tourism.

The extremes within the health care segment

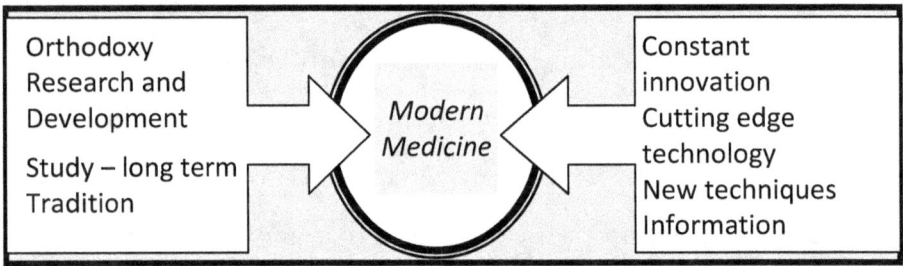

Although there are changes in the nature of the diseases that affects people, the medicine and technology continually evolves to make ever more present in the hospital environment, the process of evolution and improvement should be no different in the human relations within the hospitals. Some changes have occurred in recent years as hospitals are not anymore perceived as a cold and sad place, the health care can be warm and the human relations still be restricted to the professional field if desired.

The hospitality services significantly reduce the tensions of patients and their families at critical moments of pain and weakness, helping to restore the dignity and making possible the patient/client meet their needs. Despite the recognition and value placed by patients and visitors to hospitals that invest in hospitality services, the vast majority of hospital administrators seem to show no interest in humanizing the care provided to patients. The understanding of what is to humanize the care varies greatly from one professional to another within the healthcare industry and in the same hospital.

Features of comfort and luxury services
inside hospitals

To provide differentiated services for special customers considered VIP (Very Important People) in hospitals, it is important to go beyond the cosmetic changes normally seen in some institutions. Initially it is important to differentiate what kind of clients the hospital want to focus, creating an internal segmentation to guarantee that expensive services will not be delivered to ordinary customers, and important clients able to change public opinion receive no special attention.

Some services may be extended to all customers, while others are intended for certain groups or to a highly select clientele. Some products and services can be universalized within the hospital structure due to gain in scale and become an important tool for promotion and marketing for the institution. Others may need to be directed to exclusive customers due to high costs as the provision of items of famous brands, rooms with larger dimensions and expensive amenities.

Among the products and services that may be offered or made available to customers are:

• **Gastronomy** with differentiated meals enhancing the smell, flavor and visual appearance. The ideal is to have a customized menu daily printed with choices to make possible the patient choose their preferred food every morning.

• **Chefs** working with nutritionists and physicians in the creation and composition of the dishes.

• **Laundry room** for guests use. Obviously not the same equipment used for the hospital. It is an internal business unit, or use a third party service picking-up and delivering the clothes.

• The **outfit**/material used in the suites need to be differentiated, such as Egyptian cotton and famous brands.

• **Room Service** 24 hours with varied menu, serving patients and families who wish to be served in the rooms.

• **Religious assistance**. It is important to have some contact with all possible religions, phone numbers, addresses, times, and if possible the name of a contact who can respond by the faith 24 hours a day.

• **Concierge** or a **hospitality team** making daily visits to all clients.

• **Hair dryer** in the bathrooms or for lease.

- **Flat screen TV** (over 32 inches).

- **Cable TV** or satellite music channels in all rooms.

- **Wi-Fi**, with notebook or tablet renting services at the request of the patient.

- **Amenities** of famous brands such as Hugo Boss, Dior, Givenchy, etc. or partnering with national brands according with each region or country.

- **Robe** for patients, even if for only those at the most expensive suites.

- **Magazines** and/or **newspaper** - preferably from the region or country of the patient.

- Partnership with **hotels** in the surrounding area to facilitate access for patients and caregivers before and after hospitalization. Hospital staff can evaluate important factors in the hotel as room size, ease of internal movement, additional services offered, distance from the hospital, etc.

- Use of **wood panels** covering medical equipment. Embedded

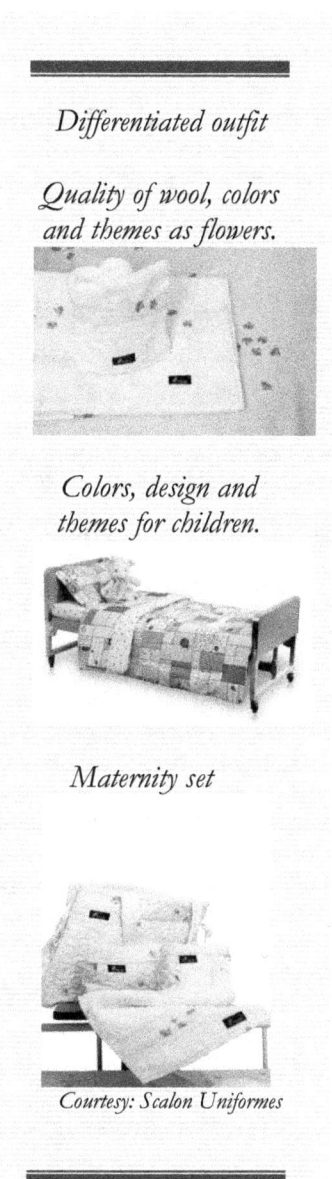

Differentiated outfit

Quality of wool, colors and themes as flowers.

Colors, design and themes for children.

Maternity set

Courtesy: Scalon Uniformes

furniture with items such as refrigerator, TV screen, music system and other devices.

• Use of **technology** such as the inclusion of equipment in a single control, use tablets and netbooks for registration and consultation of medical records and patient information.

• Provide **virtual visits** without predetermined times, sending flowers, messages and virtual cards any time.

The arsenal of resources for the hospital to differentiate their services is vast, as the discrete and alternative access for patients like authorities and personalities who do not wish to appear in the media. Some solutions are intangible, but with a big impact on the structure of the services, as the time spent on discharge in which the process is often time consuming considering the time between the physician information and patient discharge. Taking good care of the patient, will let him loyal, always choosing to return where he feels safe and well cared for, even if the doctor leaves the institution he will return to the place he trust. Better yet, will talk about the services with more people and attract attention and more patients.

The importance of hospital architecture

Architectural features very common in modern hotels, like boutique or design hotels can be adapted successfully to hospitals.

Even if the image transmitted may look too modern or too farfetched for a hospital. Several books show how the hospital architecture has evolved in many countries, especially in the United States. The hospital building goes beyond the usefulness to accommodate professionals, equipments and patients, it can also be beautiful and become an icon or a reference in the locality where it operates. Not only commercial buildings can be architectural references in many cities, hospitals may also be perceived through other images that go further than the conservative and romanesque pattern.

Dr Esther M. Esternberg in his book "Healing spaces: the science of place and well-being", published by Harvard University Press (2009) reports the importance of hospital architecture as a way of contributing to the cure of the patient in less time than usual. She quotes a study published in the Science Journal in 1984 which showed that patients was recovering much more quickly when they were in rooms with outside views, especially natural areas.

The study conducted by Roger Ulrich aimed to analyze how the outside view through windows in the hospital rooms could contribute or not to the recovering of the patient. Patients were monitored throughout the time involving all sorts of possible tests as electrocardiogram, blood pressure, temperature, etc. Were selected 46 patients, thirty women and sixteen men with common characteristics and similar surgical procedures. Twenty-three patients were placed in beds with view to the window where trees could be seen, while the other twenty-three had their beds facing the wall.

Was recorded all vital signs of patients and other health indicators, including dosage of medication, medication to control pain and length of hospitalization. The study was limited to 46 patients, due to they were within the study pattern such as age, sex, smoking history, previous hospitalizations and surgery. Even the care, was taken by the same healthcare professionals, permitting Roger Ulrich to have control over the variables that could affect the recovery. As a result, patients who had a view of the nature required fewer doses of strong medications for pain, as well as they were discharged one day before the other group of patients. Roger Ulrich was the first to measure the effect of the environment in the recovery of patient's.

Interestingly, some tropical countries with plenty of natural sunlight does not utilize this natural light as others countries with a long and rigorous winter. The light is associated with life and good feelings, causing a change in the mood of someone when he comes out from dark and enclosed environments to enlightened ones. Also increasing the interest in the life and creating hope for a person when he is sick. Previously, many hospitals were built with a structure that allowed them to take maximum advantage of sunlight, including the now common solariums where patients could absorb the healthy daily sunlight.

Although the architects strive to build comfortable hospital buildings with modern installations, still do not favor the needs of patients and their families. The spaces are created and decorated according to the perspective of the professional who idealizes or according to the needs of the managers, hardly counting on the participation of professionals who care for patients and could decide on the best way to structure spaces. The old adage that "a picture is worth a thousand words" may have its truths, like a beautiful building with marvelous services helping the professionals do their job, patients feel healthier and visitors feel safer.

%	Staff feelings after going to the hospital garden
80	They felt calmer, more relaxed, less stressed, happier
33	They felt more energy, stronger
22	They felt better, with a positive mindset
22	As an escape from the desktop, the work space
8	For religious motivation
5	It helped to better reflect on their problems
3	The time passed quickly
3	Have not affected the mood

When addressing the urban and vertical hospitals, usually located in densely populated areas with no room for traditional gardens, the sky gardens become the most appropriate answer to solve the problem. Building gardens in front of the rooms with flowers and plants of small size will create a good impression in patients who can see flowers and pay attention to small details that usually go unnoticed to the citizens of big cities.

As difficult as it sounds, you can see birds and butterflies over the hanging gardens of some hospitals in urban areas. The position of the bed in relation to the hanging gardens creates an excellent viewing angle for those who are lying. Often it is only in moments like these that many people are fascinated with a single drop of rain that flows slowly through a leaf till drop, or even realize how beautiful is see the sun among the plants. Sounds simple, but can make a difference for a patient to fight fiercely for his life or rest quietly into the death.

The gardens can even be built on existing structures in older hospital buildings as they face a retrofit, being inserted in the external walls without compromising the structure of the building. As the drawings below shows, the horizontal gardens help to preserve the view from within to the outside with the plants partially covering the view for those who are lying. While the gardens reduces the exterior view without sacrificing natural light, creating a false wall with small steps with or without plants keeping the primacy of sight.

The model with inward inclination is an excellent alternative for areas where the environment is not very pleasant, with much noise, have other buildings too near and construction sites reducing visibility inside, and avoiding that the patient have unpleasant glimpses or may look just the walls and other building windows.

Horizontal gardens: the outside view is unobstructed

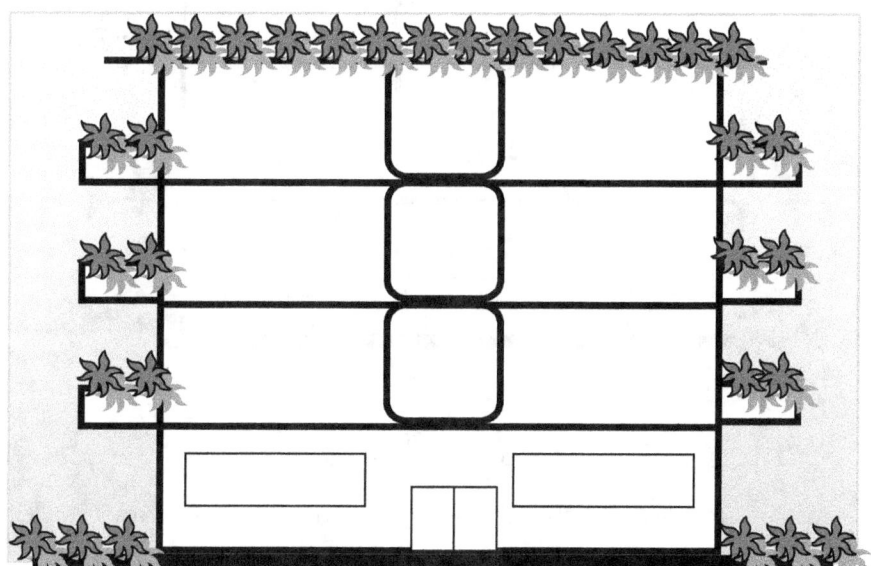

The technique is not new and historical records show that it has been used since the hanging gardens of Babylon. Questions arising about the possibilities of doing such change in buildings have been remedied with projects carried out in old residential buildings at cities likeNew York, Paris, Sao Paulo etc., which has received big balconies valuing the place without compromising the physical structure of the building. Building gardens is much simpler than large balconies.

Inclined gardens: the outside viewing is partially obstructed

The goal is to create a green oasis even where there is apparently no room for traditional gardens. To paraphrase an old adage, if you cannot take patients into the garden, then you should bring the garden to the patients. Engineers and architects should never overlook the power of how these changes can influence the patient and family perception within the hospital environment. The use of colors, water fountains and plants act differently in each person and can have a restorative effect, as well as, calming and relaxing effect with others. Even if it serves only to decorate the environment, it worth's the investment to make it more pleasant and humane the hospital structure.

Transform the hospital environment will result in other intangible benefits not always calculated for those hospital administrators who see more costs than benefits in these changes. A change in the environment is also a change in the attitude and behavior of people who come to appreciate the new space and building architecture. Moreover, these changes end up being used as marketing tools for hospitals that do not hesitate to show their buildings surrounded by gardens or isolated in a blurred image or surroundings.

Some buildings are beautifully flowered in springtime, changing the business image of the hospital building. The picture below show a small building with a few floors with garden

Hospital with horizontal gardens

The plants are in front of the large windows on each floor, creating a sensation of been surrounded by a garden, even in the middle of a busy district, creating a better atmosphere.

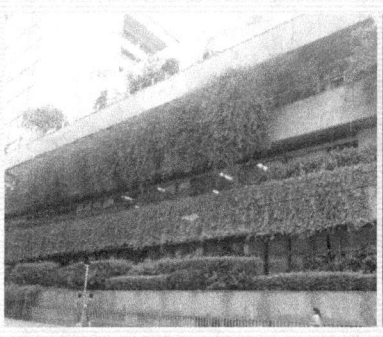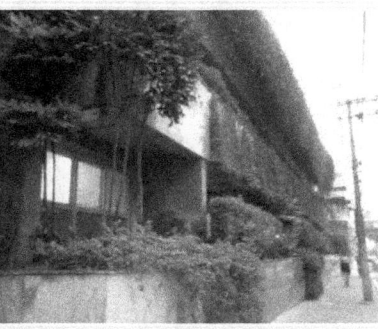

window, but this can be used at hospital buildings with many floors.

The contrast between the tense internal environment of a hospital ends up being replaced by the quiet and relaxing atmosphere, the external environment with gardens provide, especially when they flourish attracting birds and butterflies. Obviously the garden must be well maintained, if possible with flowers and be accessible, there is no advantage to have beautiful gardens or places no one knows and that cannot be used.

Healthcare institutions can take advantage of green spaces in different parts of its facility, not just as a scenario, but as a useful and resting place. The initiative can be associated with sustainable actions extremely important to the environment such as recycling, reducing the consumption of paper, water, electricity and other depletable natural resources, even seeking certifications such as LEED® (Leadership in Energy and Environmental Design).

As normally occurs, what is innovative today or in some instances will become a requirement in the future. The firsts to make the changes may even face challenges and higher costs, but will receive the biggest bonuses for pioneering. And, as happened in other countries with this trend, many institutions in the industry is seeking quality certifications and looking for to be environmental responsible. Maybe it does not happens by direct pressure of consumers, but can be necessary to renewal contracts, obtaining financing and negotiating with the major health plan operators better premium payments.

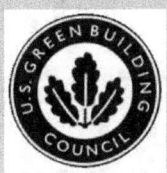

LEED® - *Leadership in Energy and Environmental Design*: is a certification system that evaluates and certifies sustainable practices to reduce the impacts of buildings on the environment. It was developed by the Green Building Council in the United States.

Chapter 8

THE ADVANTAGES OF
HOSPITALITY AT HOSPITALS

Our modern society has seen a significant portion of its productive force in all sectors of the economy, be victimized by new or even old diseases, and the growing resistance of some virus to conventional medical treatments. Spending on public and private health represents a considerable amount of income of the country, and mainly personal incomes for those willing to pay for quality medical care, despite prevention efforts worldwide.

Unexpected situations such as epidemics or endemic diseases, accidents and higher crime rates can increase a demand for medical and hospital services temporally or definitely. Not citing the regular demand, sometimes letting private and public hospitals working beyond its normal capacity. All this has a high social cost that the society has no way out to escape, paying sometimes for the precariousness of the services offered to citizens, because the demand is far superior to the existing capacity.

On the other hand, technology and recent advances in medicine have provided accurate diagnoses to patients and a cure much faster with a shorter hospital stay, although many by virtue of its clinical severity remain long periods hospitalized. Compared to previous decades there was a significant improvement in health services worldwide, especially in the underdeveloped countries. But, what about the hospitality practiced in these hospitals, the importance of humanization in the hospital environment and how it affects the service as a whole in public and private hospitals?

Initially we must make a clear division between humanization and hospitality in hospitals. Both are converging, but there may be individually very different environments. Although the hospital may have excellent hospitality services it does not make it humane, and may even have five-star hotel services, and have very little human warm with their clients. Similarly, humanized hospitals may not have necessarily an infrastructure of hospitality that differentiates it from the competitors. Although the ideal is making these two worlds working together, but not always is possible to join them.

What is it? The hospitality in hospitals aims to introducing techniques, procedures and hotel services in hospitals with the consequent benefit social, physical, psychological and emotional to support patients, families and hospital staff. The humanization is the action to humanize care, making it sensitive to the needs and desires of patients and families, through actions that aim to positively transform the hospital environment, understanding it in all its moments.

To create hospitality services is necessary to invest a minimum of financial resources for purchasing equipment, hiring employees and implementing new services. To humanize is on exclusive dependence of human actions, motivated by unselfish concern of changing the internal hospital environment for the better. Thus, hotel services in hospitals are usually associated with private hospitals, which may also be constrained in public hospitals, whereas the humanization does not necessarily depends on financial resources, exist and can be worked anywhere. Of course, the private institution still enjoys the ease of working both variables if desired.

Defining hospitality services as one of the goals of the institution

The human attendance in health care industry had improved in recent years, as a result of investments in training, technical skill improvement programs, quality focus and other factors as the increasing competition among hospitals, which made them aware of their competitors. Moreover, the hospitality treatment should not differ greatly from one hospital to another, as in fact occurs in many places and countries.

Because of their nature, hospitals are still seen by most people as a cold and impersonal institution. There is a gap in the relationship between the client and healthcare professionals, there is no emotional involvement that may compromise treatment, in many cases the professional create its own wall of protection. It is a kind of security fence for some and protection for others. Furthermore, the risk of infection, infectious diseases and the death are part of the daily routine of these professionals creating an invisible distance or barrier, which is often a shield to guarantee that personal feelings may not be involved.

The daily care of the patient involves pain and suffering and can change the personal and collective feelings of a significant number of professionals, who care directly for patients. A physician-surgeon can not necessarily feel sorry for doing a surgery with a high risk of death in one patient, when this may be the only alternative to prolong or save the life of a patient.

Although the decision is often up to the patient and family, but the doctor will not leave untouched emotionally the operating room if the results are not the best. He is also a human being who also feels and suffers. However, while in some situations the emotions needs to be restrained, in others it is unnecessarily, especially when the human being who works in a hospital can become part of the remedy for clients and family.

Here we have a dichotomy: the existing technology in hospitals, the accumulated technical knowledge and improved physical structures against the hospitality and care dispensed to patients in most hospitals, with few exceptions. Hospitals are complex institutions to be administered and despite their efforts, there is sometimes lack of infrastructure improvement and humanity, making the treatment less traumatic to the patient, making the hospitality staff as agents of warmth in contrast to the common cold hospital environment.

The hospitality can reduce significantly the suffering of customer healthcare especially in moments of emotional pain and weakness. There are many isolated initiatives coming from institutions with consistent success and bilateral benefits to those who engage in these processes. However, these initiatives have been timid and cartesian, involving only one or another department and does not cover the entire universe of action within the hospitals. With them the hospital takes a new image, that is not just to treat disease, but to produce knowledge, quality of life and sell your main service, health.

In general, the concern for the welfare of human beings during a hospitalization should start even before the hospital begins to work. Because the architecture has a fundamental role in the hospital, the project needs to replace stairs with ramps and elevators, have open spaces ventilated and lighted course, gardens and green areas reduce the stress of patients during hospitalization, differentiated and/or reserved entrances and exits facilitates the movement of patients within the hospital when they need to be taken to other departments during the treatment and so on.

Some architectural successful projects even managed to replace the air-conditioned, by taking advantage of natural ventilation air currents of the locality in which they are based. The involvement of architects and engineers with the staff and healthcare professionals who will use the spaces is of fundamental importance for the project to be functional for those who will use it, from the client's health to the staff and visitors. (Rogar, 2002)

The existence of services previously devoted exclusively to hotels in a hospital facility, allows minimizing the inconveniences generated by a hospital, as anxiety and emotional distress that ends up involving the family client's health. Another effect felt by the hospital is the increasing demand for higher quality services, even if it means to bear higher costs. Normally the consumer ends up choosing a better service, even when it is more expensive or when their life or the life of a loved one is at stake.

Hospitality means that the hospital is very close to the services of a hotel, with a clientele with different needs and with a much higher degree of sensitivity to the environment. Therefore, aggregate services offered at hotels make the recovery less traumatic and less stressful for the client's health. Some hospitals have already made it a daily reality, including the staff, hospitality managers, housekeepers, chefs, concierges, among other professionals who permanently changed the concept of quality of care in hospitals.

Services previously unthinkable as a porter or doorman, came not only to bring more comfort to customers who arrive at the hospital, but also acting leading the front door services, preserving the cleanliness of external areas, caring for the safety of those who arrive by an attentive view of the surroundings and close contact with the security department, among other duties common to catering. Couriers or bellboys works assisting in the arrival of customers and visitors, taken them to check in, help while in the apartment and later in the discharge. They also help various demands like flowers, gifts, papers and others patient needs while hospitalized. Providing services and enable a smooth transition of all patient stages is a great merit that the hospitality brought to hospitals.

So, on arrival at the hospital the client is warmed welcomed by the porter and have his car parked by a valet, while staff helps with its luggage leading them to check-in, and then to the apartment explaining how to get the various services offered, as well as proper handling of equipment. This is also one of the advantages of the hospitality service at hospitals. Many hospitals are investing in valuable equipment to customers, but did not have professionals who assist them to use properly, reducing the rate of breakdowns and maintenance of such equipment. Check-out follows the reverse procedure resulting in complete assistance to client and his family. The impact of initial and final services, sometimes creates a greater impression, bigger than many events during hospitalization.

The visual impact caused by the new structure also includes new hospitality spaces like small shops with gifts often forgotten or not taken to hospital, as flowers shop, coffee shop, small art gallery or small museum, hair space, among others offered by the hospital. To offer such services minimizes the effects of a prolonged hospital stay by offering something that could cause some inconvenience if do not exists. Although there are the same services outside the hospital, the offer within makes the stay of clients, family and caregivers less painful, and also serves their own employees, when there is no ban by law in the country.

Restaurants can be as warm as they are in other places. Food also need not to be restricted to bland menus, the menus may be appropriate to high cuisine and prepared by recognized chefs, bringing more flavor to the taste of customers and staff. For clients, better to be at home than in a hospital, but if you have to stay at least the food should be more pleasurable. The focus now should be on what the customer can eat, not what he cannot eat. This is a change of mindset in hospital gastronomy.

The apartments can be tastefully decorated, while continuing with the usual equipment such as oxygen under wooden panels. It is possible to find several models that are discrete and take up less space than the older models. Working on color therapy really has a calming effect on the patient (chromoteraphy). Supply comfort items such as LCD or plasma TVs, refrigerator, waiting room, amenities with items known or by famous brands, and some occasional pampering left on the bed like a card with a message of encouragement from administrative staff, doctors or nurses, some candy (if allowed) or even a newspaper the customer likes, can make some difference.

Although the hospital does not necessarily need to build customer loyalty to stay running, some customers are interesting to the organization and need to be treated with more attention by the department of hospitality. In many cases, little pampering can make a big difference. For example, is common the client forget the sandals to move indoors inside hospital, which can be offered by the hospital. Some customers are highly profitable generating a high bill, and the hospital can give a robe during his stay. The impact will be minimal in the patient bill. It is a gift that can be taken home and can have on its inside lapel hospital emergency phone numbers. It's the kind of gift that hardly anyone refuses, and can be delivered only once, or one by year.

While addressing the hospitality, the offer of amenities has been common in almost the majority of hospitals. Agreements with famous brands, may result in providing these amenities pampering guests, promoting the brand with differentiated customers while the hospital benefits from customer satisfaction. It is important to emphasize that marketing departments of many companies spend large sums advertising in the media, whereas such measures make a positive propaganda for free by the institution.

The hospital does not thereby become a perfect place to stay, but facilitates the recovery of human dignity, attending to their needs in the critical periods of its life. These are ways to humanize the care provided to these organizations, which with the offer of an improved infrastructure, constant training of professional and customer-focused health, improves the care provided by making him feel important and owner himself, having respected his space, having his body not treated as an object, and especially being taken into account their emotional characteristics. (Lopez, 2002)

Empathy seen since the initial care by first contact (marking procedures, getting insurance authorization, etc.), a quick check in preceded by a warm welcome, a respectful treatment tends to cause a deep and abiding impression that tends to be durable in the mind of the patient. The very permanence of the patient in the hospital need not be fruitless during hospitalization. After discharging may attend concerts, lectures and theatrical performances when the hospital is fitted with appropriate spaces. Computer, stationery and pen on the room table may result in stimulating the client to write to loved ones, or develop some text to let your impressions of those moments.

The activities may turn not only to patients due to the difficulty to engage them or create specific activities for them, as also for companions and visitors who are often distressed and anxious, they need ways to let the tensions escape. Especially when they are accompanying prolonged hospital stays. Develop internal activities and open to the participation of a larger audience, such as lectures, plays, music concerts and musical performances tend to have a calming effect and allows a temporary escape from the problems that surround them.

For hospitalized children, groups of clowns or actors which simulate medical actions has proved invaluable to alleviate the suffering of those who sometimes cannot even understand why they are there. Although there is still resistance from these professionals in the hospital environment, the vast majority have accepted them without any problems. Despite recognizing the importance of the beautiful works like these, it is disheartening to note the lack of interest there is in hospitals administrators not conducting similar studies. It is worth mentioning that the simple use of music in some areas, produces a wide range of beneficial and relaxing feelings for customers, visitors and the employees themselves. (Revista do Incor, 2002)

Implement changes that improve the quality of services provided, which makes the structure more appropriate to patient care and also meet satisfactorily the companions results in increased customer satisfaction. Which will express that to the employees who feel gratified by working in an organization that enjoys respect in society and the medical community, generating increased demand, resulting in increasing revenues, constituting a virtuous circle whose tendency is always growth.

Although the purpose of the client stay in a hospital is the medical treatment, this set of additional services from the hospitality department becomes a valuable complement contributing to the medical treatment. The attention to details and professional interest in reducing errors and failures, transform the critical moment of contact with the patient, exceeding their expectations, and offering differentials that will take effect on the final evaluation of the client about the institution.

Future prospects for hospitality in health care services

The hospital is one of the most complex human organizations ever conceived. Managing it is a difficult task given the many variables involved, as well as Peter Drucker pointed out in an article in Harvard Business Review (2002) Journal. There are more than thirty areas of management with professionals from various specializations necessary for their operation, and a large contingent of employees from various fields. Is administered the work of an assistant or a gardener with low formal qualifications, while others have PhD titles or international recognition. Some may be dispensable while others may be considered indispensable to the institution. Various inputs, medical teams, laws and rules, policy's, economic environment, insurance health plans, and finally, there are a lot of people which makes necessary attention to every detail.

Although participating in many different ways, everybody is essential in a hospital. Not only is the human capital, the most important asset of a company, but the fact that the care provided to a client from these professionals, impacts in the final perception of the services offered by the hospital. Although efforts for a good service are usually centered in front-line staff, they too often face problems when they do not have the properly support inferring in the final result. It is important to strengthen a culture that not only who meets the client needs to provide good care, who is working behind the scenes is also an internal customer, acting together with others working on the frontline.

A customer will not be well served if the one who serves does not have all the tools and structure to do so. Another major factor is the autonomy that people who work in key areas need to have to solve small daily problems. Delegate is still something that needs to be learned for most of the leaders, often with unreasonable fears, still not delegating, often punishing strictly any deviation occurred, as if it was not a natural consequence of professional learning. It is not uncommon for leaders to circumvent or disappear in the face of common problems with clients, reappearing later when the situation has "cooled" seeking to know what was done or looking for someone to be blamed. This spread a climate of insecurity and uncertainty among staff, which is usually reflected in the quality of the work done.

To work the hospitality effectively, is needed to follow the job done by the departments involved in the customer service and from others who support them. Eliminate the internal feuds, where each department has a cartesian view of its activities, regardless of what the next department is doing is vital for the processes to be holistic. In some cases, it is advisable to encourage visits from one department to another to encourage the exchange of information and increase awareness of how a problem in a particular department can affect the other creating a chain. Some of the activities that result in the hospitality services depend on physical processes and steps, not just smiles and warmth at the time of service. A friendly smile is of little value if the problem of a customer is not resolved.

To implement the hospitality is not just putting a porter at the hospital door, hire some bell boys and remodel the apartments. It is a philosophy of care that goes beyond physical and structural changes, need to permeate throughout the environment and everyday life of the hospital. This is a process that involves structural changes in the building and equipment, which is the easy part, it is also necessary other educational process that may take several months or years, the hardest part, needing to be made by all the professionals of the institution as a change of mentality in client care.

You may need to drop some paradigms in the health segment, which still persists in perpetuating unhealthy models of blue hospitals, cold and impersonal at all. It is common the resistance to new concepts of quality when they are introduced into the area of healthcare, which may require caution in its introduction, not enforced or as an obligation, incurring in the risk of failing in the face of resistance, widespread apathy or antipathy.

Changes often cause fear, therefore need to be managed properly so that does not result in rejection. Among the ways to deal with these situations, is the effective communication, transparency of actions, because people normally fear what they do not know well, and knowing can contribute to the improvements. Also, creating an atmosphere that encourages the involvement of everything, to highlight the benefits that everyone will have a new and better image in the market.

Changing the hospital environment and humanizing the care provided has been the goal of sensitive administrators who realized that they cannot sell just the medical treatment, anymore. The ordinary medical treatment is a commodity. It must provide an additional structure of services, in many cases necessary to restructure departments and implement changes before unthought. The implementation of hospital catering services in part or in its entirety, appears to be still difficult for many managers who feel afraid to deploy it. Or for those who already have some services, but are afraid to implement improvements because would entail additional costs, or even the fear of distortion of the hospital image.

An increasing number of hospitals is looking for to modernize its structure bringing modern concepts from architecture or hotels to renew the hospital environment. The result has been attracting a qualified demand able to pay more for additional services besides the medical treatment. Sometimes, the media exposure and also the change in the image of the hospital in the market pays the investment. To other hospitals, there will be enough to compete for the same market without major differences

Improving the hospital services

The market has always offered more functional and modern equipment to facilitate the work of healthcare professionals, and make the stay of a patient less painful in the hospital rooms. Just take a look at the medical equipment's a decade ago and compare them with currents, is possible to realize how significant the changes have benefited everyone. Large hospital fairs held every year have focused on specific areas as hospitality in hospitals. New furniture with various shades, colors and shapes with a modern look combining the design, comfort and ease of use by patients and caregivers are created every year.

Equipment such as automatic beds allow some patient autonomy, and more peace of mind for caregivers and nursing professionals who no longer need to make great efforts to change its position. Even the dining table received new items that make it less uncomfortable to the patient's personal hygiene when walking to the bathroom is compromised.

Many hospitals have used the color therapy as part of the changes implemented. Others have changed the trousseau of pediatrics units using children motives like cartoons in the uniforms used by the professionals who serve them. Providing wireless environments or points of Internet access in the apartments has been useful for those who want or need to maintain some contact with the outside world during hospitalization. There are hospitals that provide tablets or laptop computers for patients who do not have or did not bring their personal equipment to the hospital.

Additional equipment such as small refrigerators has been helpful to patients and caregivers, as well as flat screen televisions with cable TV programming, although it is considered common items in hospitals. Personal hygiene products are usually delivered in small sets that can be branded and famous. Both benefit. While addressing the improvement of the structure to support caregivers, has been common stores for last minute needs, flowers, a space devoted to the beauty, space for leisure and comfort where public musical performances occurs.

The cuisine has also been one of the aspects that have greatly improved in recent years. Previously the focus was on what the patient could not eat, today is exactly what he can eat. Except when necessary, menus with multiple options are common to those who are hospitalized bringing a little more flavor to bland hospital food. For caregivers and other professionals restaurants have been a pleasant environment where families can talk comfortably while they wait for their meals or medical information.

Many patient companions notice suddenly they are in a strange city and sometimes less safe than where they live. Providing maps and information is helpful when the stay is prolonged. Professionalize the information provided by the staff in the corridors about where to go and how to get something, avoids trouble and gives more peace of mind for the visitor. It does not mean having to always have a concierge, but a proper brochure supplies or the material on the internet. (Andrade, 1999)

Before focusing attention only to the internal public hospitals also produce and distribute knowledge through courses and other events. The use of auditoriums and internal infrastructure enables events to be performed by generating revenue and serving the purposes of the institution as training, specialization courses and other events specific to the area of health such as conferences, forums, seminars and lectures. Some institutions have developed nursing courses and expertise in various areas of healthcare. Where knowledge is produced, can also be multiplied and made available to other professionals who will benefit doubly, the course itself and the practice of running a hospital, differently from the theories that educational institutions commonly provide.

The spaces can be renovated and cozy, providing moments that minimize the suffering caused by hospitalization to patient and visitors. Musical performances by small orchestras, choirs, theater presentations, presentation of musical groups, lectures of public interest, art exhibitions and other activities can be developed in pre-determined dates and communicated to all clients.

A major problem in hospitals is that they are not always designed and made for patients and their families, but for healthcare professional's work. There are many obstacles and difficulties that hinder movement of patient beds or with wheelchairs. Open areas with natural light, bright colors in public areas or with large circulation, airy windows that allow views of gardens are invaluable for those who need to move through different places whose walls are all equal and the rooms do not differ a lot from another.

When planning the installation or restructuring departments, such as an intensive care unit (ICU) should be thought of situating them in areas with gardens view, parks or green areas. Although it may seem a utopia in big cities, small gardens can be suspended. Only those who are terminally ill or hospitalized in critical condition know how much it means to see a bird sipping water in a flower, imagine the smell of wet leaves or the scent of a flower and see the leaves swaying in the wind. These are small shows that the nature provides and people have no time to notice before because of the routine, but the eyes of a dying man can grasp.

These little gifts and surprises from nature can restore the strength to fight against the death or to struggle in search of life that may gradually fades or be the reason to rest in peace. Been one reason or another, to live or allow itself for a smooth eternal rest. At least can be considered better than dying in front of a TV, with the cold air conditioning, among lights on day and night, the noise and lifeless colors of an ICU.

There is much that can be done to improve the hospital structure, but still depends on an attitude and willingness to be daring and creative in the hospitality offered to consumers of health services. The watershed of quality has often been the time when members of senior management or when medical staff are hospitalized, so they see how the service and structure can be improved. This perception allows the provision services that make more human or can guarantee the dignity during treatment, precisely at times when the person is more fragile and required to submit to a medical intervention.

The hospitality offers a comprehensive range of options that focus on the consumer of health services as the main benefited in difficult times when their health is poor or the life is at risk and may result in death or disability. To train and educate employees to be good listeners, encouraging them to be understanding and helpful can greatly alleviate the suffering caused by lack of normal family life in such circumstances.

Good care is one of the main factors determining that the patient feel welcomed and their recover may occur in the shortest possible time. Empathy and psychological support will reverberate throughout the physical and mental convalescent making him feel like the only one during treatment and contributing to the stay seems shorter, although it occurs in the same space of time that is necessary.

The implementation of hospitality projects

A good project of hospitality and/or humanization can be developed within a hospital successfully, if some details are perceived and observed carefully from the beginning. Since the commitment is essential, one should not disregard the involvement of any professional throughout the process. From the cleaning staff to the director, everyone must participate and contribute when possible. As we know even those who do not meet the customer must bear in mind that are supporting those who serve.

Like any project, there will always be people who agree and disagree with the means the hospital adopts for the results to be achieved, many of which will show explicitly faults and deficiencies of people and departments that will certainly result in discomfort and resistance. Others may disagree with the changes because there are still those who believe that the hospital must have the "hospital smell" and have "to seem like a hospital." Even respecting the diverse points of view, there are changes that need to occur, being or not being accepted.

To help, the technology can play a vital role with computerized systems for real-time information that bring flexibility in attendance and promptness in solving problems. Tablets and smartphones have been extremely useful with softwares that tell the manager in real time the daily amount of funds generated in procedures, tests and hospitalizations, including providing information about specific account that is stopped at some department exceeding the pre-determined time to be charged.

Unlike what is commonly imagined the hospitality department does not work only the human side or humanization, involves technology used in all equipment in the apartments, also the furniture, colors and ambient sounds in the various departments of the hospital, infrastructure and services that involve from the gardening to the customer service or ombudsman. As we live in a society focused on technology, this has been a great ally for the services be rendered to customers quickly.

It is possible that a client order on a floor is immediately transmitted by mobile equipment soon after the food service professional who attended left the room, avoiding loss of time in transit procedure. The discharge process itself can be optimized with the customer early access to the account on the TV's own room or smartphone message. Similar to electronic medical records, requests for different patients can be stored for future reference as special foods, favorite newspaper and peculiar habits.

Bringing flexibility in attendance, problems of transition activities may be evident, as well as problems of communication and relationship between people and the various departments involved. There is also the need for familiarity with the technology, which is not always possible in hospitals with very old employees. Problems related to the organizational culture that is relevant in organizational behavior, may hinder the implementation of deeper changes consistently.

For the process to be effective, even with professionals averse to change, it takes them to participate actively as peer educators, encouraging their teams to invest in the new format of care. This means to monitor the managers to ensure they are aligned with the objectives expected. Many managers do not understand clearly what is expected from them, others do not in fact contribute to the changes, there are still those who explicitly agree in a meeting and disagree internally not encouraging his staff to participate effectively.

One way to develop the activities is to turn it an educational process, divided in stages or phases to be measured and monitored. To be effective it must:

• Define what the focus or interest of the institution/hospital: investing in technology (software, programs, smartphones, etc.), physical infrastructure (furniture, modern equipment, etc.), services or humanization;

• Determine what resources and/or investments are necessary and available;

• Establish goals and/or phases to be achieved by pursuing periods each not too long (from 3 to 6 months each);

• Develop an efficient system of marketing to disseminate the activities;

• Involve all employees. Even the associates or service providers.

It is possible to plan the development of activities in three phases according to a schedule, that may be established by the project team responsible for the activities.

Phase 1 - Dissemination of activities

Possible division into sub-phases:

- Campaign for clarification of its importance

- Encouraging the participation of everybody through marketing actions

- Encouraging the development of department activities jointly with company aims

- Assessment of needs and available spaces

- Etc. (e.g. fundraising, partnerships, investments, etc.).

Phase 2 - Training of human resources

Possible division into sub-phases:

- Training all human resources involved

- Acquisition of equipment and materials

- Development of a sense of team and importance through courses and actions

- Adequacy of the spaces to the proposed activities

- Etc. (e.g. in-company courses, professional training, hiring, etc.).

Phase 3 - Deployment / Implementation

Possible division into sub-phases:

- Moment of truth (putting into practice)

- Adaptation to the needs aroused

- Search responsiveness with customers

- Discussion of expectations and results
- Perception of services by employees (through research)
- Feedback of results to all involved
- Etc. (e.g. re-adjustment of the project, implementation of improvements, etc.).

For all activities to be successful and the involvement of all, sometimes is necessary to remind them the professional valuation in the market when the hospital is in evidence. The compromise produces tangible results that enhance the image of the hospital and therefore the professionals working on it.

The hospital management with focus on hospitality services

As a natural process, the world is undergoing a constant and nonstop change. Each society adapts to these changes in its own way by creating new patterns of behavior or adapting others to the new ways that appear every day, many of whom come from meeting the needs of various segments of society. These changes often generate new requirements to meet the new systems resulting from these changes. These needs require new staff or re-qualification of existing staff to meet the aroused demand. These professionals develop activities and actions that result in environmental changes affecting the system again and restarting the cycle. The image below shows the sequence of social changes brought about by the changes in the market behavior.

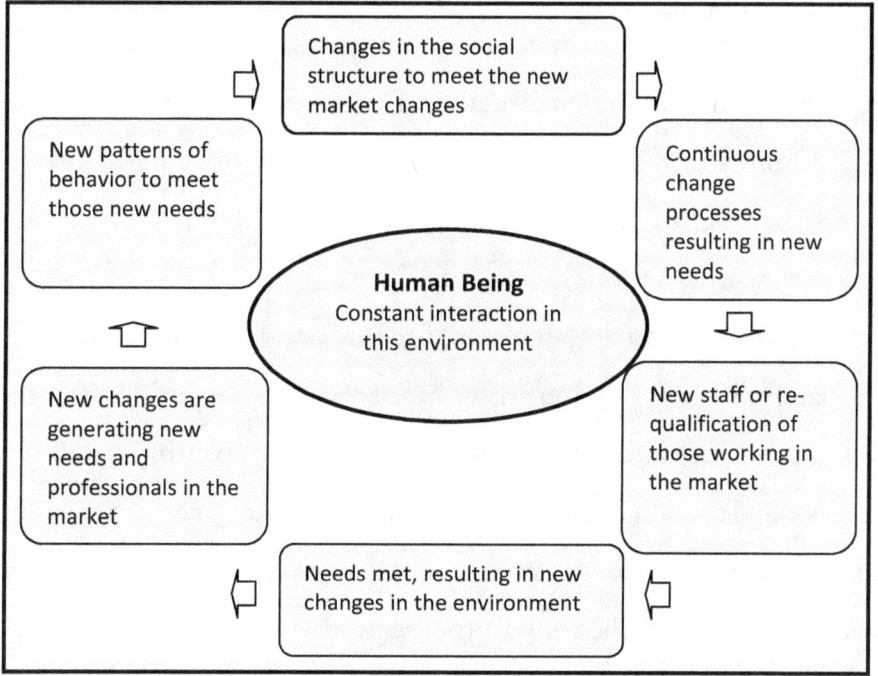

One of the most perceived changes that have occurred in recent years, was the improvement in the quality processes within hospitals. With more information available and awareness of their rights, clients realized that they may require services that meet their needs, even when dealing with subjective matters. Aspects, before related only to medical procedures and outside the administration scope of work, have become part of everyday life of the administrator, even coming to their attention through channels such as the media or Customer Service.

Although the hospital administration is still characterized by conservative patterns of management; usually contrasts with the innovation and technological advances of the industry, such as new techniques and medical equipments, which is part of the work environment. The difficulty of inserting new behaviors and new administrative trends in hospitals is still resistance, among other reasons, for fear of spoiling the hospital environment with new management models.

Many hospitals lately assumed a new posture focusing in the patient's recovery and in its human capital, especially for the patients whose attention must be given as a priority, and not necessarily the "doctor" as is usual in many countries. The modern manager needs to fit or adapt to new trends that are emerging and consolidating in the healthcare market, deploying or implementing services or changes in humanization, or running the risk to face competition, sometimes from the other side of the world with better and internationally accredited hospitals.

Although hospitals have a captive demand, because they would never miss patients in face of increasing demand for health services and preventive care, it does not mean that patients drawn are exactly the stratum they want. New hospitals have emerged in recent years with a different proposal of services, while others invested in the modernization of its structure and improved the hospitality offered to their customers. As a result end up targeting different portions of the population that require added services to medical treatment and are willing to pay more for it. The insurance companies and health plan operators are aware of the demanding for these services and attentive to the calls of their customers. Others that are stuck in time or moving slowly, will remain disadvantaged and lose the opportunity to increase the price charges to insurance and health plans.

It is significant that the hospitals needs to act decisively in the pursuit of continuous improvement of services they provide to their customers. This improvement may occur with a joint effort conducted with partners and suppliers, especially the insurance and health plans operators that are closer to the clients and know what are the main problems encountered in hospitals. The operators themselves may require improved services to pay more, and also can conducting regular courses to fit professionals to national and international standards of quality services.

The deployment of hospitality services and the development of humanization actions need to enter in the plans of managers who wish to maintain their hospital competitive. The costs of the investment often return in different ways, with improved services and increasing the qualified demand. Moreover the image of the hospital will be strengthened in the market resulting from a positive advertising usually generated by the exposure in the media. These changes should be qualitative requirements when health insurance plans start operating in the hospital.

Create or design strategies that will meet the real needs of customers, or to produce a differential before other companies, will make a good manager with its employees achieving the goals that must be the same of the company. Encouraging teamwork with each professional continuing the work of the previous professional and team, from the client's arrival to discharge, in other words increasing the systemic work with input, processing, output and feedback has proved advantageous, as should be natural in the hospital environment.

One goal of modern management is to predict future risks and opportunities of a company's business. The manager should remain alert to the possibilities of new business and improvement actions that may arise internally, not just waiting for expensive consultants hired to say what many professionals already know inside. Many of the problems existing in the companies are known by its employees in the department where they occur, and even their solution. Perhaps, employees do not know how to structure a solution or implement it properly what managers should do, because they have the training and position to do so.

Many improvements have not even given, due to the staff knowing or fearing that the credit will not be given to them.

Surveys with clients involving regular exams, hospitalization and the emergency care, can be a barometer of how the care is provided in the hospital. Old clients can opine how the hospital has changed in recent years and how these changes were perceived. Data interpretation is also of paramount importance, many times the complaints of poor hygiene and cleaning may be associated with poorly painted walls, torn uniforms and unkempt appearance of some employees. It is easier for a customer to realize a piece of paper on a clean floor, than see a clean floor with a piece of paper. A good job of after-marketing (even sampling) can bring to attention some situations not perceived day-to-day, bringing excellent results at the end.

A hospital manager alone could hardly stick to all the details and problems, or even be aware of all the improvements that may occur in the physical infrastructure and the human needs. It need to surround himself with competent and committed professionals. To empower their staff to implement changes, even with the proper monitoring of the direction has been difficult today in the healthcare industry.

Many managers want to control all the changes in the institution imposing its own way of managing, pruning professionals who innovate or have a sharper future vision, resulting in a reactive institution. Everybody knows that top professionals and improved care in the hospital will increase significantly the demand due to the superior service, sometimes not due to the manager. Since this is a change of mentality in an industry averse to rapid innovation, the recovery may be slow and costly, in view of the rapid scrapping of hospital equipment and defaults caused by leakage of talent for competing hospitals.

Managing the patient satisfaction

As happen in all business relationships, not always the hospital-client relationship is healthy all the time, occurring some dissatisfaction, complaints and even lawsuits, although the rule observed is satisfaction. When the problem is with the doctor or nursing staff, very few complain afraid of retaliation or face problems with the staff, as many prefer to do, look for another hospital and another doctor. Although it is an industry that is unlikely to feel the lack of customers, we could feel a reduction in the desired segment and worse, the attraction of unprofitable new customers.

Clients and families in the age of internet are increasingly aware of their health problems, rights and options in the market. It has been increasingly common lawsuits to repair damage or securing rights, either against doctors, hospitals or insurance plans. To stay tuned to the hospital-client relationship, open to meet the clients and hear them, and paying attention to the service quality delivered, can reduce the problems that lead even to lawsuits.

The existence of good ears in departments as customer service allows clients to feel safe and supported upon the occurrence of some internal problem or doubtful situation. In some countries the society itself has created a bad image of who complains against any care or service, resulting in the search to other service or to find another hospital than to face a slow and exhausting complaint process. In practice there is a drain of precious resources to other institutions that offer similar or better quality service, even at a higher cost.

In developing countries still prevails the divine role of the physician (or a so called physician-centrism). Their verdict is absolute and unquestionable truth, not delegating to the patient the right to decide what treatment they want to follow or giving the treatment according with his convictions, and not necessarily the possibilities existing in the segment. The treatment ends up being imposed despite the secular consent from, who have no options (Mezomo, 1995).

There are also family members to resort to some doctors for more information often received with distaste, getting answers in a hurry, evasive, with technical language, vague or imprecise.

Usually these physicians are not bad professionals, but because doctors cannot give the luxury of dispensing more than a few minutes to their patients due to strenuous routines and care in different hospitals.

In moments of sorrow and regret every word of a doctor can be weighted and give rise to different interpretations by the relatives of a patient in critical condition. The physician and writer Moacyr Scliar wrote "***Every word spoken by a doctor to his patient is a verdict. As the writer, it should evaluate each word and know how to use it with extreme rigor.***" Another major factor in treatment is to take care of the soul, spirit and not only the body, the physical appearance. As quoted by Buchalla in the same text, "... the lack of technology and resources are offset by long and affectionate conversations. Sometimes that's all the patient needs." (Buchalla, 2004)

While we see an increase in technology used in hospitals, we also see an increasing distance between doctor and patient. The personal contact even professionally who values human relations has been reduced every day, especially when trust between the patient and the hospital should be maximized throughout the treatment. The high investments in technology and medical equipment, does not always mean improvement in diagnostic results or the accuracy of them, this information is currently undervalued, even by those who thinks that the more modern hospital, the more reliable it is.

Administrators and physicians need to know how to analyze the resources they have, investing in what is essential, but not forgetting the human side of the business. Strategies that value older concepts that never ceased to be modern, as treating the patient's body and soul, and with the time gave way to abstract conjectures, need urgently to change. (Caravantes, 1998) There is a need to open discussion between doctors and administrators, and especially the government's attention to one of the most important areas, the health care, and for the professionals in her heroic act, be treated better.

A new support structure for employees

Problems exist in any organization and the vast majority of them goes unnoticed by the board of directors or even comes to its attention. However, many of these problems are small thermometers of great value for many different internal evaluations. As is natural for its strategic position, the manager turns to macro indicators' neglecting much of what occurs in the lower levels that are indicative of larger problems that hatch later. Large fires start small with a short circuit. The service area that has direct contact with the customer and who experiences the moment of truth all the time, is often neglected despite isolated efforts of some professionals. At the end of the administrative pyramid is natural that the customer contact is reduced and the information coming suffer distortions of what actually happened, because usually go through several management filters.

Professionals working in direct contact with the client in hospitals should receive ongoing support in the form of courses, psychological support, relaxing activities and still have an anonymous communication channel directly to the board. These are professionals who are more prone to mood changes and bad temper of unstable clients and those who compensate for flaws in the structure if any, is the human service that makes the difference, and they deserves investments as well as those done with technology.

The nature of the hospital structure is horizontally oriented (Drucker, 1999), not allowing large internal drives as a nurse who may be a manager, or a doctor who becomes a physician team leader, and so on. This creates many difficulties in maintaining the provision of professional growth within the hospital, or even to retain highly talented professionals. As one of the most complex human organizations exist, the hospital needs specific policies encouraging working professionals to work with a new approach, to preventing or minimizing the monotony of lack of prospects for professional growth. Among the alternatives used there is a horizontal movement with use of professionals in other departments of the same hospital and internal replacement programs, beyond the now traditional vertical mobilization.

To streamline the work and produce better results is the possibility to implement physical activities such as fitness as a routine, as part of the daily activities of those working directly with clients and visitors, or even indoors, as a means of relieving tension and let these professionals more calm and peaceful. The gymnastics or short breaks throughout the day with light exercises can quickly reduce the burden of daily tensions.

A gym inside the hospital or agreements and partnerships with gyms near the hospital, with theaters, clubs or other leisure facilities, or the introduction of a professional to act internally, can produce all kinds of positive results. Regular physical activity for employees have been recognized by specialists and verified by managers as a way to reduce health problems, reduction in turnover rates and raises individual and collective productivity. Other consequences such as, increased attendance at work and increased sense of importance, are factors that can be perceived. (Buchalla, 2002)

Of great importance in the hospital environment is the dominant mindset among healthcare professionals that will define the environment in which they operate. The new prevailing mentality is that the hospital does not exists only to treat health problems and sickness, but *"to sell health"*. Health is the main product or service sold by hospitals. All other values are aggregated to it. The daily life of those who work in hospitals puts professionals in touch with the constant pain and suffering, though many moments of joy. The situations experienced every day can severely influence some practitioners reflecting on their actions inside and outside the workplace. Knowing that the "health" is the main marketing product that the hospital has to offer its customers should be clear to everyone in the hospital environment.

A new dominant mindset can significantly alter the outlook for future growth of the hospital, including the perceived effort and satisfaction among the employees themselves. The consumer of health services that have options to choose, prefers to identify itself with a hospital service which is geared to meet quality and institutions with a positive image in the market. Even for professionals in the healthcare industry, it creates an expectation and competition that attracts the best people for these hospitals. Everyone wants to work in centers of excellence no matter the area or position to be occupied, is a receptionist, administrator or doctor creating a virtuous circle, with excellent professionals improving the hospital which in turn will attract more and better professionals.

The supportive structure provided to patients

The quality of facilities and accommodation the hospital offers largely determines the customer profile attracted by the hospital. Much of the conventional medical treatment has been commoditized and can be found almost anywhere in the world, so comfort and quality of the structure offered by the hospital took a new and greater importance, because the health client's not only wants to be treated, he wants to be "treated well". The room is the space where the patient will remain most of his time, allowing greater opportunity to improve the care than commonly spent. The use of the wide range of services will make the stay more enjoyable, or at least have a less painful recovery during hospitalization.

As part of the support structure can be deployed some services such as concierge, where from small and basic to big needs the customers and their companions can found without incurring unnecessary risks in a strange city, as a beauty space, shuttle service, lodging and meals. Some hospitalizations are prolonged and the family does not cease to live, visiting museums, theaters, doing sightseeing and enjoy shopping.

In other cases patients and visitors arrive days before the hospitalization and travel days after the discharge, having to wait some time in the city, which ultimately results in complementary activities to treatment. To whom it may seem strange, the hospital is a place where people of all ages, fields and professions meet, resulting in interesting business relationships and even marriage. Some hospitals even perform marriage ceremonies between clients who met during hospitalization.

Partnerships with mourning companies for difficult times, given the high degree of complexity involved with the documentation, especially in transfers to other states and countries in cases of death, reduce the sense of abandonment of the clients who feel vulnerable when they are in strange places. Employees who deal with these moments need to be properly trained to understand "the moment" of the family. Many try to be polite with ready-made phrases or religious messages that generate even more problems. It is unusual for employees to be trained to understand the habits and customs of people in situations such as grief, which leads to misinterpretation when witnessing acts of mourning people from different religions.

Other services that are available and of a great help to family members and even for internal staff of the hospital, are luggage locker and couriers, being useful for internal and external staff. The medical information is not always clear or always available, and is also a source of problems for the hospital itself, especially in broken families. It must have a formal system of information to family members and in case of hospital authorities and personalities through verbal and written medical reports, each appropriate to the situation that is inserted. Establish ways to ensure effective communication between doctor and patient is as important as the management team to clarify the correct functioning of its structure to their staff.

Although there are routine medical visits, is increasingly common complaint from customers that, the doctor even looked in his eyes or knew his name. Interestingly, customers rarely complain directly to doctors for such problems. As the nurse makes a visit to every patient at the beginning of their work, the same should occur with the doctors. May be only five minutes, but will be five valuable minutes of confidence infusion. For each customer is very important to know not only from their own doctor, but the name of the doctor who is responsible for the unit where it is admitted at that time. This information only conveys a sense of security and proximity to the medical and nursing staff, even if no intervention is necessary.

The external structure of the rooms and corridors also need to be rethinked. Professionals from other fields such as hospitality, architects and designers can change markedly spaces for public or common use. The use of bright colors, modern artwork, paintings on walls, plants and gardens where possible enhances the lightness of the environment by bringing more peace and quietness to those who work or are passing by the hospital. Some hospitals put spaces recovery as physiotherapy and hydrotherapy in front of gardens and woodlands. There are hospitals praised worldwide for use of natural lighting, rounded shapes and even natural ventilation in indoor areas where this is possible. (Rogar, 2002)

The internal service supply, restaurant or room service with a high quality of services and products offered are departments that deserve management attention. Many people at hospitals do not have or have few dietary restrictions, which enable the food service along with the responsible physician to make compromises when possible. Not everyone in the hospital are patients, there are physicians, families, visitors and other professionals who work or are developing some other activity also looking nice places to make their meals. In addition, customers who usually go to fancy restaurants see sometimes forced to eat a bland food unnecessarily because there are no many possibilities on the menu at the hospital restaurant. Chefs have increased the menu of many restaurants and made delightful this basic human need, even within a hospital. (Moherdaui, 2001)

Although there is still a great rejection by some communities, it is widely known the virtues of complimentary therapies in the treatment of some patients. A few years ago it was unthinkable to bring an animal during a patient convalescence, which today is highly encouraged for the recovery of many patients and certain types of diseases (Veiga, 2007).

Since 1800 (in England) the animals began to be used successfully in medical treatments, known as Animal Assisted Therapy resulting in numerous successful projects in hospitals in several countries (Zaché, 2004). Among other ways adopted is music therapy and participation in manual activities (patchwork). Very different than some might imagine, many are prone to new treatments that can alleviate the suffering and indicate possible areas of improvement.

Provide a vehicle to receive customers at airports, do a city tour or take them shopping may seem closest to hotels than to hospitals. However, with the increased arrival of medical tourists becomes important to create an external support structure to their needs, which involves including the hiring of guides speaking other languages, and booking tickets for theaters and cinemas. Customers who arrive from other regions have the same needs as foreigners and also benefit from the same system.

Spaces such as lounges and VIP lounges are useful to accommodate personalities and be used as an area intended for press/media during interviews, and can offer things like quick massage to different customers. Buffets, breakfast or afternoon tea service can be both provided to family and visitors using the restaurant in alternative hours. Conservatories and solariums make the environment more pleasant making the hospital climate mild and more acceptable. Among the business units underexplored in some countries the hotels are attached or belonging to the hospital to accommodate family members, visitors, healthcare professionals and even the general public. In case of non-viability of this business, partnerships with hotels allow more affordable and safer accommodations for customers.

The vast majority of hospitals prioritize the amount of beds and not always the quality of the space where they are, as occurs in intensive care units (ICU). The beds usually stand side by side with each patient observing everything that happens with the patient to the side or in front, even emergencies that lead to deaths.

It is not easy to describe the fear of a person who is fighting for his recovery, see another person die at his side or in front. Partitions can obstruct vision, but not necessarily the running professionals taking care of who will fight for life at risk. Witnessing moments like these let the adrenaline high in healthy people, much worse for the convalescent who is subject to similar situations. The contact with the patient next should be allowed only if desired by both, which is already possible with movable or removable rigid dividers.

These units tend to be collective and cold for obvious reasons, but some changes can humanize the permanence of those who are in it. Individual units, individual controls for lighting and windows overlooking gardens or landscapes where possible are of great help. In large urban centers where open spaces are rare, suspended gardens outside, the chromotherapy among other innovations could mean a lot for patients. The rustle of leaves (even inaudible), birds that sip water in small water fountains, flowers in gardens may be the reason that a patient needs to fight so fiercely for life or rest quietly in peace. Innovations like these will allow a manager absent or distant realize the importance of these changes, instead of the cold numbers over his desk.

Hospitals and clinics that offer a differentiated and a high quality service have given rise to a new customer profile in the market, as well as a new philosophy of service to the public that the environment affects the healing process, and increasing comfort and confidence in relationship between the client and the hospital. As a result there have been comparisons and an increase in demand for these services, improving the concept taken from the hospitals and significant improvement of satisfaction among customers.

However, the conservative view of many managers, despite their competent performance has limited the actions within hospitals discouraging initiative and been affected by the company culture. It is a wide range of possibilities for new services, even restricted to centers of excellence, which could be developed within hospitals with large financial benefits to the organization, improvement of professional qualification, low implementation cost and higher quality of services offered.

It is up to senior managers to analyze the extent possible of all possibilities presented to a hospital company to create or promote activities, new products and services to meet their goal which is to rescue and/or produce health. The modernization of the hospital cannot be restricted to modern equipments. Knowledge is also an important part of the investment in technology and involves professionals who work with the most perfect of all equipments, the human body. Analyze the entire environment in a holistic manner anticipating the changes, will enable the manager to obtain a significant return on investment in a market that is increasingly aware of their needs and desires.

Cultural and leisure activities at hospitals

A sudden hospitalization is no longer a reality as far as it was some time ago. Accidents, violence, new diseases or health problems that affect the humankind and the gradual deterioration of health due to senility, may force us to a hospital for medical treatment that may be brief or prolonged, affecting the physical and emotional sense of a person. Moreover, with advances in medicine and increased life expectancy, more people have sought preventive services previously diagnosing diseases that in other times would cost their lives prematurely, allowing achieving a cure and getting less painful and aggressive treatments as in the case of cancer. Except for preventive situations and even with more hospitals and clinics, the increase in health problems has led to a consequent increase in the flow of patients seeking the public and private hospitals saturating care.

Be withdrawn abruptly or scheduled from within the family, work and social activities, has a profound impact on emotional and psychological aspect of human being. Whether by accident or disease, it is an extremely difficult time for the patient and their family members, when vulnerable require too much attention and sympathy during this difficult time. This is one reason why the institutions that care for life, should make every effort in order to rescue the patient health and give him back the joy of living. Not only treating the disease, but taking care of the patient as a whole, physically, emotionally and psychologically.

One way is by starting changing the mindset of employees and physicians, encouraging a healthy view of the hospital as a company that sells health and life, offering possibilities of recovery from diseases. After all, the hospital consumer product is "health", that's why it exists is to sell health, to return the patient to a healthy status. But to occur, a series of measures need to be taken, ranging from the marketing strategies to bring patients to the medical follow-up after treatment.

Due to the length of time the patient remains hospitalized at the hospital with the sole occupation of a television, the time can be filled with activities provided if the patient clinical condition permits and the environment are ideal for it. Some recreational activities and entertainment can be performed within the hospital facility, making shorter the period of convalescence, although they occur with greater intensity in the wards of pediatricians and to elderly people.

The companions and family can enjoy regular lectures on topics that the hospital see interesting made by the hospital staff such as doctors, psychologists, physiotherapists, nurses, engineers and others professionals. The family members will become enriched and can share their experience when returning to the room with the patient. (Lopez, 2002) The hospital shall also provide something that produces constantly: knowledge and distribute it paid or for free, like courses and specializations that already occurs in teaching hospitals. Themes can address obesity, posture or other topics related to human health. When possible, some patients with good medical condition may also participate, providing an emergency support if needed.

With prior permission, the patient can get volunteer's visits for a few hours or even minutes for a nice conversation. Some hospitals use volunteers to make visits to their clients gathering information about the service in general, however, to be genuine must be altruistic. The situations that show the importance of human contact can be realized with the patients that are little visited, although he or she has a large and wealthy family.

Once, the call operator of a hospital warned the hospital manager of the night shift, about an unusual amount of long distance calls from a room of a patient in chronic state of its disease. When investigating the situation, he was discovered that the rich old lady with no prospect of cure, was calling and making bidding in expensive jewelry on a television program in an attempt to spend her money, as she found herself abandoned by their always busy family. Of course it was reported to the right hospital department to deal with this situation.

Such situations are not uncommon in private hospitals aimed at upper-class customers. On special occasions like birthdays, Christmas and New Year eve, there are families that make everything possible to keep their parents as long as possible at the hospital, sometimes complaining against the patient's discharge. The hospitality department can increase the perception from the channels available to identify customers in unpleasant situations and provide a differentiated service.

There are hospitals that already have its own theater group, formed often by employees and involving all departments.

The presentations occurs at various times and special occasions to the hospital, mainly focusing children and in pediatricians. It is impossible to describe the satisfaction of a child when in contact with initiatives like these. A playroom in a hospital can be, sometimes, a piece of paradise on earth if the children can go there. As many doctors will say, it will not cure the disease, but will allow some moment of joy and alleviate the pain in the way only a child can explain. Do you still have doubts? Ask a child under cancer treatment!

Choir presentations or musical groups have also become common in many institutions. Something to be avoided is to restrict the presentation only to professionals in the organization. Visitors, associates, relatives and in some cases patients with medical permission can also enjoy these magical moments. It is well known throughout the health system, how this can change the environment resulting in the patient satisfaction. The changes in the mind and body influences directly the psychological side of the patient, causing an improvement in their health when is a way of escape from the tension while hospitalized.

To visit some pediatricians in hospitals can be painful and difficult task, many children even do not fully understand their suffering and why they need to be hospitalized. And they do not stop being a child during hospitalization and the treatment. Except for a few moments of relaxation of a visit, very little is allowed to those who suffer silently without knowing how to express their pain and feelings.

Recreation rooms or playrooms cannot bring back the child's health or reduce the length of hospitalization, but may return in a few moments the happiness of being a kid again. The child does not cease to be a child while he is ill and has no cognitive conditions to fully understand what is happening with their body, being necessary to compensate the pain and suffering with activities that make them forget about the environment they are. (Oncken, 2002)

Such activity may consume more time from everyone in the hospital, can generate some investments and result in some costs not scheduled. It will demonstrate the social responsibility of the hospital with the society. What really will be worth the efforts and investments will be the many smiles, laughter and good memories despite a bad period, these children can receive treatment with one of the best remedies known, the human warmth.

To introduce leisure and cultural activities in hospitals, we need to understand the human side of people, to make less stressful and traumatic the stay in a so strange home. Although for some people the hospitals are a home or almost a second home, due to constant and long stays and hospitalizations. Lopez (2002) discusses the difficulties of the patient and family that are in the midst of the unknown and unexpected, especially when they are even more fragile finding the coldness and pain in attendance instead of the warmth, attention and respect.

The activities may involve regular visits by volunteers to donate their time, whether in private or public hospital, professional artists can donate their time teaching techniques as folding (origami), for patients and caregivers during their hospitalization. It's a job that has no end, because there is always a turnover of patients. Clowns can visit patients weekly, especially those children in cancer institutions. Toys and games could be donated to fill the free time of many young patients facing treatments. And books could be found largely in all wards, to guarantee an opportunity to fly away from the hospital while lying in a bed.

Another essential factor is the permission of the patient and his family for the activity, whether an adult or child. Without permission, no activity should be authorized by the hospital or should occur. A basic principle is to respect the time and pain of the patient. Unfortunately, there are hospitals that refuse the offer of artists and other professionals who want to donate their time and skills to make visits to hospitals.

The hospitality department in private hospitals can work distributing gifts during visits, or even giving a newspaper or magazine at each visit. Hospitals that have libraries can make their books available for loan to families and caregivers and patients, taking care not to make the book a disease vector. In hospitals where the hospitalization is prolonged, if authorized by the physician, activities can be developed with visitors and family. An injured young patient, who faced a hard time while in treatment after an accident in the city of Rio de Janeiro (Brazil), tells one of its rare moments of leisure in a public hospital.

> *When we got back to the male ward, we joined in a group to play cards, the only fun activity at night. The cards were much worn and I made a mess because I could only move my right hand to hide cards on the table. I immediately thought of asking my mother to bring my playing box with chess and the game War. When I asked the colleagues if they were interested, they cheered. They had no money to buy this kind of game, they considered from elite, but liked to play. (Lucena Junior 1998: 124).*

Obviously the reality is different at every hospital, the same way is the positioning of health professionals about these subjects. Like many clowns in hospitals are rejected, animals are still considered incompatible with the hospital environment and complimentary treatments are viewed with suspicion because of lack of scientific basis, many refuse to accept humanization initiatives in hospitals. Many professionals believe that a hospital is a hospital and will always be a hospital, and needs to look like a hospital.

The recovery period during hospitalization allows the patient to have enough time to indulge in various activities that usually take the time he usually doesn't have, but that may be useful or generate pleasure, like reading, chatting, playing games and discussions when possible about themes that the short free time of the day-to-day life does not allow. The hospital itself can help stimulate the use of time for these activities. It should be activities available without any obligation of acceptance and without compromising the treatment. The results can be difficult to quantify, including the moments of evasion or avoidance that clients and companions will enjoy.

That is it. To make every moment of life worth, to have the best and safe treatment possible, to enjoy hospitality services and get humanized attention when hospitalized. It should not be a differential, but an ordinary routine at hospitals. If it is not today in all hospitals, will be in the future in those places who care for ill people. I hope all professionals can change their mind, not when they also face a hospitalization, but trying to see that all industries are giving out their best to keep their customers. It should not be different at hospitals when we more need it. It is up to us to change, and not always wait someone change something. Make a difference! If not in yours, make in others life!

REFERENCES

Almanaque do Luxo. Veja São Paulo edição especial. Revista Veja ano 43, n. 46. São Paulo: Editora Abril, novembro de 2010.

ANDRADE, José V. Turismo: fundamentos e dimensões. 6ª ed. São Paulo: Ática, 1999.

AQUINO, Ruth de. É hospital. Mas pode chamar de hotel. Revista Veja, São Paulo, nº 15, ano 35, ed. 1747, pp. 84, 17 de abril, 2002.

BUCHALLA, Ana Paula. Check-up: você ainda vai fazer um. Revista Veja, São Paulo, nº 16, ano 36, ed. 1799, p. 83, 23 de abril, 2003.

_____. Doutor, me ouça. Revista Veja, São Paulo, nº 18, ano 37, ed. 1852, pp. 85, 05 de maio, 2004.

_____. Médicos ditadores. Revista Veja, São Paulo, nº 36, ano 35, ed. 1768, pp. 11, 11 de setembro, 2002.

_____. Malhação capitalista. Revista Veja, São Paulo, nº 31, ano 35, ed. 1763, pp. 66, 67, 07 de agosto, 2002.

BOEGER, Marcelo A. Gestão em hotelaria hospitalar. São Paulo: Ed. Atlas, 2003.

BUCHALLA, Ana Paula. Doutor, me ouça. Revista Veja, São Paulo, nº 18, ano 37, ed. 1852, pp. 85, 5 de maio, 2004.

Caderno de informação da Saúde Suplementar: beneficiários, operadoras e planos. Ministério da Saúde. Agência Nacional da Saúde Suplementar. Rio de Janeiro, dezembro de 2010.

CARELLI, Gabriela. Entre a vida e a morte. Entrevista. Revista Veja. 10 de agosto, 2011. Páginas 17-21.

CASTELLI, Geraldo. Hospitalidade: na perspectiva da gastronomia e da hotelaria. São Paulo: Saraiva, 2005. Contas satélite de saúde do Brasil: 2005-2007. Série contas nacionais nº 29. IBGE, 2009.

CARAVANTES, Geraldo R. Teoria Geral da Administração: pensando & fazendo. Porto Alegre: AGE, 1998.

COSTAS, Ruth. O turismo do bisturi. Revista Veja, São Paulo, nº 3, ano 39, ed. 1940, pp. 88, 89, 25 de janeiro, 2006.

Dicionário Brasileiro de Língua Portuguesa. Jornal da Tarde. São Paulo: 1996.

DRUCKER, Peter F. Desafios gerenciais para o século XXI. São Paulo: Pioneira, 1999.

DRUCKER, Peter F. Eles não são empregados, são pessoas. Revista Exame, Harvard Business Review. São Paulo: Ed. Abril, 2002.

Folha de S. Paulo. Saúde. Maioria dos prontuários médicos é mal preenchida, diz pesquisa. Quarta-feira, 26 de janeiro de 2011, C10.

DANIELOU, Jean & MARROU, Henri. Nova história da igreja. Petrópolis: Vozes, 1966. v. I, pp. 131.

FERNANDES, João. V.; FERNANDES, Filomena M. V. SPAs, centros talasso e termas: turismo de saúde e bem estar. Lisboa: E. Pergaminho, 2008.

FUSTER, Luiz Fernandez. Teoría y técnica Del turismo. Madrid: Ed. Nacional, 1974. t. II, pp. 567.

GODOI, Adalto F. Hotelaria Hospitalar e Humanização no Atendimento em Hospitais: pensando e fazendo. São Paulo: Ed. Ícone, 2004.

GODOI, Adalto F. O Turismo de Saúde: uma visão da hospitalidade médica mundial. São Paulo, Ícone Editora, 2009.

GRAHAM-POLE, John et al. Restoring lives, restoring selves: The arts and healing. International Journal of Arts Medicine. Volume IV, n° 1. Saint Louis/MI-USA.

HAJJAR, Ludhmila A. et al. Transfusion Requirements After Cardiac Surgery: The TRACS Randomized Controlled Trial. Journal of the American Medical Association. October 13, 2010, vol. 304, n° 14, pages 1559-1567.

Humanização no atendimento. Tendências. Revista do INCOR. São Paulo, ano 7, n° 72, pp.16, 17, 2002.

Institute of Medicine. To err is human: building a safer health system. Washington (DC): National Press Academy, 1999.

LEAPE, Lucian; Lawthers, Ann G; Brennan Troyen A., et al. Preventing Medical Injury. Qual Rev. Bull. 19 (5): 144-149, 1993.

LUCENA JUNIOR, Ricardo. Longo caminho de volta. 6ª ed. São Paulo: FTD, 1998.

LEEBOW, Wendy (ed.). Service Excellence – The Customer Relations Strategy for Health Care. USA, AHA, 1988.

LEPARGNEUR, Hubert. (org.). O enfermo: Perspectivas pastorais. São Paulo: CEDAS (Centro São Camilo de Desenvolvimento em Administração em Saúde), 1987.

LOPEZ, Immaculada. Doente também é gente. Revista Problemas Brasileiros, n° 354, ano XL, pp. 16-19, Novembro/dezembro 2002.

Manual internacional de padrões de acreditação hospitalar. Rio de Janeiro: CBA: UERJ, CEPESC, 2003.

MARCUS, Clare C; BARNES, Marni. Gardens in healthcare facilities: uses, therapeutic benefits and design recommendations. The Center for Health Design. CA/USA: Eusey Press, 1995.

MEYER, Philippe. A irresponsabilidade médica. São Paulo: Ed. UNESP, 2002.

MEZOMO, João C. Gestão da qualidade na saúde: princípios básicos. São Paulo: Ed. Metha, 1995.

NAZARETH, Janice C. Poderemos, enfim, novamente morrer em paz! Visão Médica. Hospital Alemão Oswaldo Cruz. Ed. 07, maio, 2011, pp. 29.

MAIA, Jayme de Mariz. Economia Internacional e Comércio Exterior. 9º ed. São Paulo: Ed. Atlas, 2004.

Manual Internacional de Padrões de Acreditação Hospitalar. 2ª ed. Rio de Janeiro: CBA: UERJ, CEPESC, 2003.

MASETTI, Morgana. Soluções de palhaços: transformações na realidade hospitalar. São Paulo: Palas Athena, 1999.

Medicina Defensiva. Em defesa de quem! Debate. Revista Ser Médico. Ano IV, nº 21, Out/Nov/Dez de 2002, pp. 24-32.

MOHERDAUI, Bel. Tempero na canja. Revista Veja, São Paulo, nº 15, ano 34, ed. 1696, pp. 62, 63, 18 de abril, 2001.

ONCKEN, Luciana. Ayrton Senna: ação social em alta velocidade. Jornal da APM, ed. 528, pp. 20-23, setembro de 2002.

O Estado de S. Paulo. Vida. A cada 2 dias, um profissional de enfermagem é acusado de erro. Terça-feira, 01 de janeiro de 2011, A24.

O Estado de S. Paulo. Notícias. Contaminação atinge 95% dos jalecos médicos. Quinta-feira, 23 de setembro de 2010.

Padronização da nomenclatura do censo hospitalar. Série A. Normas e Manuais Técnicos. 2ª Ed. revista e atualizada. Ministério da Saúde. Secretaria de Assistência à Saúde. Brasília, 2002.

Projeto reduz ansiedade e medo em crianças antes da cirurgia. Humanização. Revista Hospitais Brasil, São Paulo, nº 27, ano V, setembro/outubro, 2007.

ROGAR, Silvia. Doutor da alegria. Revista Veja, São Paulo, nº 4, ano 35, ed. 1736, pp. 50, 51, 30 de janeiro, 2002.

SEGATTO, Cristiane. Saúde cinco-estrelas. Revista Época, São Paulo, nº 148, ano III, pp. 86-92, 19 de março, 2001.

SILVA, Maria Júlia P. Comunicação tem remédio: a comunicação nas relações interpessoais em saúde. 5ª ed. São Paulo: Gente, 1996.

SILVA, R. C.; VALIENTE, S. C. R.; BORGES, T. F.; LIMA, V. A. B.; REIS, C. Avaliação do potencial de jalecos como fonte e veículo da transmissão de microorganismos na clínica cirúrgica do Hospital das Clinicas da Universidade Federal de Goiás. VI Congresso Panamericano e X Congresso Brasileiro de Controle de Infecção e Epidemiologia Hospitalar. Porto Alegre/RS, 11 a 15 de setembro de 2006.

STERNBERG, Esther M. Healing spaces: the science of place and well-being. Massachusetts: Harvard University Press, 2009.

TARABOULSI, Fadi A. Administração de hotelaria hospitalar. São Paulo: Ed. Atlas, 2003.

The Joint Commission: Advancing Effective Communication, Cultural Competence, and Family-Centered Care: A Roadmap for Hospitals. Oakbrook Terrace, Il: The Joint Commission, 2010.

Tradução do Novo Mundo das Escrituras Sagradas. New York: Watch Tower Bible and Tract Society of Pennsylvania, 1986.

UNESP, em: Medicina de alto risco. Contexto. Revista Veja, São Paulo, n° 24, ano 37, ed. 1858, 16 de junho, 2004.

URRY, John. O olhar do turista: lazer e viagem nas sociedades contemporâneas. São Paulo: SESC, 1999.

VACCARI, Andréia M. H; ALMEIDA, Fabiane de A. The importance of pets' visit in recovery of hospitalized children. Hospital Israelita Albert Einstein. São Paulo, v. 5, n° 2, pp. 111-116, abr./jun. 2007.

Vade-mécum da Acreditação Hospitalar Brasileira. Ministério da Saúde. Revista HOSP. Editora Suprimentos & Serviços ltda. São Paulo: outubro de 1999.

VEIGA, Edison; VILICIC, Felipe. Visitinha animal. Revista Veja, São Paulo, n° 34, ano 40, pp. 47, 29 de agosto, 2007.

VIEIRA, Sônia. Hospitais cinco-estrelas. Revista Audi, n° 39, ano, 7, pp. 74-80, abril, 2002.

WELCH H. Gilbert et al. Overdiagnosed: Making People Sick in the Pursuit of Health. Boston (Massachussetts): Beacon Press, 2011.

White. S., Dillow, S. Key concepts and features of the 2003 National Assessment of Adult Literacy. Washington, DC: National Center for Education Statistics, U.S. Department of Education, 2005.

WHO Guidelines on hand hygiene and health care. First global patient safety challenge. Clean care is safer care. World Health Organization, 2009.

WHO Patient Safety Research. World Health Organisation 2009. WHO Press, Geneva, Switzerland.

World Wealth Report 2010. Merrill Lynch and Capgemni Financial Services. USA. New York/NY, 2010.

Waste Measurements. US health-care spending. Estimated waste in healthcare spending by Thomson Reuters. The Economist. Jun 17th, 2011.

ZAPPAROLI, Alecsandra, BERGAMO, Giuliana. Eles por Eles. Medicina. Revista Veja SP, 16 de setembro, 2009. Ed. 2130, pp. 32-46.

ZACHÉ, Juliana. É o bicho. Revista Isto É, São Paulo, n° 1827, pp. 54-57, 13 de outubro, 2004.

ZAKABI, Rosana. Respeite o paciente. Revista Veja, São Paulo, n° 6, ano 36, ed. 1789, pp. 11-13, 12 de fevereiro, 2003.

ABOUT THE AUTHOR

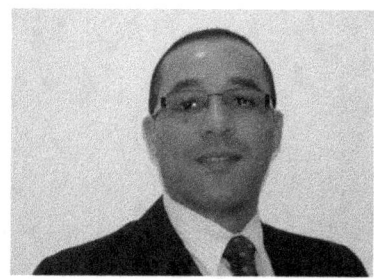

ADALTO FELIX DE GODOI

Graduated in Management by the University of London – (LSE), he holds another graduation in Tourism and Hospitality, is a specialist in Human Resources Management and have an Executive MBA in Strategic Business Management from the University of São Paulo/USP. All prestigious institutions known worldwide.

He teaches and gives lectures in some universities; works as a consultant in healthcare; is author of books and articles about hospitality, humanization and medical tourism, and has been working for more than thirty years at hospitals in management positions.